G000149248

The Case for a
Personal Psychotherapy

The Case for a
Personal Psychotherapy

Peter Lomas

Oxford Toronto Melbourne
OXFORD UNIVERSITY PRESS
1981

Oxford University Press, Walton Street, Oxford OX2 6DP

London Glasgow New York Toronto
Delhi Bombay Calcutta Madras Karachi
Kuala Lumpur Singapore Hong Kong Tokyo
Nairobi Dar es Salaam Cape Town
Melbourne Wellington
and associate companies in
Beirut Berlin Ibadan Mexico City

British Library Cataloguing in Publication Data
Lomas, Peter
The case for a personal psychotherapy.
1. Psychotherapy
I. Title
616.8'914   RC480   80-41679
ISBN 0-19-217680-3

Set by Western Printing Services Ltd
Printed in Great Britain
at the University Press, Oxford
by Eric Buckley, Printer to the University

For Sally, Jon, and Tim

What determines the direction a man
will take? Sometimes the delicate
maneuvers between his will and desire,
sometimes the heat of his vanity,
sometimes the blessing of his innocence.
But more often than not, it is all
a mystery . . . – Irving Howe, *The Decline
of the New*

Contents

Introduction

There are various ways in which an attempt might be made to
answer the question 'What is psychotherapy?' The derivation of the
term could be traced, or the meanings assigned to it by contemporary workers could be explored and compared with a view to finding
a common denominator.

In what follows I shall say what the term has come to mean to me:
therefore this is a personal book. I make no claim to startling
originality. Each of us who has a point of view that we want to share
believes it to have some originality or, at least, to be expressed in a
way that is significantly different from other writings on the subject.
I propose in this introduction to state, very briefly, those of my
conclusions I have reached which are sufficiently controversial to
require the defence I have undertaken in this book.

Most accounts of psychotherapy err, in my view, by implying a
degree of certainty in method and theory which is unjustified. It is
this certainty which – however courteously or humbly expressed –
has given rise to the appalling schisms of psychotherapy in the
present century and which engenders a proliferation of techniques
and schools of thought which is truly alarming. It is such certainty
which has allowed the work of the greatest psychotherapist of
modern times to become ossified. And it has led to the establishment of what Ivan Illich refers to as 'disabling professions'.

In the face of human misery and confusion it is not surprising that
we seek for a sure guide. In the past it was the priest, now it is the
psychologist; we follow a leader who appears to know. Without the
reassurance of his certainty we would often falter; our schemes,
whether individual or collective, would sometimes remain un-
started. But what is the price we have to pay when we accept a view
of living and of healing that is oversimplified?

Plato thought he knew how to bring up children. More recently
his successor, Dr Benjamin Spock, thought the same. And there are

psychotherapists who think they know how to heal patients. But such certainty is usually proved to have been misguided.

To say this does not, I believe, require us to take the extreme position of absolute silence. Many wise and valuable things have been said about living and healing which are well worth conveying. The objection I make is that they should not be cloaked in the authority of a system of belief which aspires to a higher form of knowledge than that available to the ordinary person. Let me give an example.

The concept of 'transference' is perhaps the richest idea that has been handed down to us from Freud. I would recommend any prospective psychotherapist or counsellor to study it with care. But if I were to make it the focus of my therapy and theory, to which all else was secondary, or if I were to proclaim that no useful therapy could take place without it, then I believe I would have narrowed my vision. I am not sure how to handle transference or to formulate it. What I am sure of is that the past has great significance for the present (that it is transferred on to who or what is there). But to hold this belief does not require me to stray from the realm of truths that come from our immediate experience and that we sometimes refer to as 'eternal'.

This line of thought will lead me to consider the balance between the ordinary (i.e. common wisdom) and the special (knowledge unique to psychotherapy); to review the importance of ordinary responses to troubled people and to compare them with rehearsed responses; to appraise the language that psychotherapists use; to consider what might be the most useful circumstances in which two people can meet in order that one may help the other (and to suggest that the essence of what we call psychotherapy lies in the circumstances of this meeting and the attitudes of the partners rather than in any theory of psychopathology); and to explore, without neglecting the lessons of Freud and his successors, the dilemma of teaching a practice which depends more on experience, courage, and imaginative open-mindedness than on anything else.

The reader who is looking for certainty should put this book down now. The dangers of uncertainty are many. Not only is it disturbing to those who seek a sign, but it presents an easy way to escape rigour and indulge in a multitude of sins. It may encourage a smug and naïve reliance on one's spontaneous, intuitive reactions,

or become an excuse for vacillation or woolliness. But that is a risk
we have to take unless we deny the enigma of life.

Let me put the matter another way. Contemporary psychotherapy proposes a framework of theory within which the practitioner may, to a certain degree, reveal ordinary human qualities. By
contrast I would suggest that psychotherapy is the manifestation of
creative human qualities in a facilitating setting, in which the task of
healing is eased by a critical knowledge of the theories and techniques of twentieth-century practitioners.

What I state here is an article of faith. I cannot prove it. It is the
best formula I can find for describing the reasons for the fact that I
can be of some use to most of the people who come to me for help.
This book is a personal testimony. A scientist would no doubt
prefer to videotape the sessions which I and my colleagues have
with patients, and try to measure the changes, if any, we appear to
effect. This is an understandable wish, derived from a scepticism
which is not entirely unhealthy but impossible to execute without
turning living into a skill which can be assessed. In lieu of such
'evidence' I present here some of the sense I have been able to
extract from my work.

Any list of those thinkers by whom one has been influenced must
be arbitrary, and much is a matter of chance. I am sure I could have
been educated less painfully. The impact of Freud is decisive and
obvious. But in my departure from Freud – and from science –
which constitutes much of the impetus for writing this book, I have
gained especially from the work of Henri Bergson, Martin Buber, John
MacMurray, Ludwig Binswanger, Erik Erikson, Charles Rycroft,
Donald Winnicott, and those (Lidz, Bateson, Wynne, and others)
who first called our attention to 'schizophrenogenic' families. Jung
should, of course, have been in this list but, alienated by much of his
writings, I failed to appreciate his worth until I had reached this
position through other paths. I have also increasingly come to
realize that the urgency of my opposition to the prevailing view of
psychotherapy is part of a long tradition in philosophy, one that I
recognize in the description by Hausheer as an expression

of the great battle begun by Hamann and Herder against the central values
of the eighteenth- and nineteenth-century faith in liberal rationalism,
cosmopolitanism, science, progress and rational organisation . . . and
continued in the twentieth (century) by existentialists, anarchists and
irrationalists, and all the varying strains of contemporary rebellion and

revolt. For all their deep differences, these thinkers, groups and movements are brothers beneath the skin: they fight in the name of some direct,
inward knowledge of self and free causal agency, and an irreducible sense
of specific concrete identity.[1]

From time to time in this book I shall describe my experiences
with those who came to me for help. I know that these descriptions
are bound to fall far short of the actuality, and therefore mislead as
well as reveal, but my belief in the 'irreducible sense of specific,
concrete identity' has provoked me to make the attempt.

References

1. Hausheer, R. (1979), Introduction to Isaiah Berlin, *Against the Current*,
   Hogarth, London.

1. The Question of Wisdom

I am strong. I cultivate in myself the best human
sentiments: love, devotion, honesty, abnegation, heroism,
disinterestedness . . . – Avdennko, addressing the Seventh
Congress of Soviets in January 1935 (quoted by David
Caute in 'The Illusion')

In what is called 'individual psychotherapy', two people meet and
talk to each other with the intention and hope that one will learn to
live more fruitfully. In spite of significant variations, this, in general, is the form it takes. How can such a thing happen? How can one
person help the being of another?

Firstly, and most obviously, someone may be expected to help by
means of his wisdom, love, sympathy, strength of character, and
whatever simple virtues that will avail in his efforts to bring succour
to the one in distress.

Secondly, a person may help by measures which are out of the
ordinary: by invoking powers derived from supernatural sources, or
by the use of techniques which, under the influence of the scientific
tradition, have been gathered together by specialists into various
theoretical frameworks and methods of working. Because I am not
concerned in this book with the supernatural (for I have nothing
useful to say about it) my discussion of this second kind of help will
be limited to the scientific approach.

I want to make it clear that I am using the word 'technique' in this
context to denote that form of behaviour towards another person
which derives from a special body of theory. I therefore differentiate it from 'tactics' or 'strategems' which, although often referred to
by psychotherapists as 'techniques', are, in fact, simply the kind of
ploys which we use in ordinary life, and are a manifestation of an
attitude which (if we approve of it) we call 'tact', or (if we dis-
approve) we call 'manipulation'. The confusion between the words
'technique' and 'tactics' has, I believe, arisen because those who
rely on a body of theory inevitably take a detached view of the
therapeutic encounter – a view which has something in common
with that of the person who, in ordinary circumstances, has a
tendency to adopt a tactical approach to people rather than act
spontaneously.

It would seem possible, and perhaps likely, that this similarity is not accidental – that it results from the fact that people who are reflective and cautious in their relationships are drawn towards theory more than their fellows. Therefore, while making the distinction between wisdom and scientific technique we may note that the extent of the gap between the two depends in part upon our ideas about wisdom: if we consider that a wise man is shrewd and circumspect we will expect him to take a detached if not 'scientific' view.

It is as well, I think, that I lay my cards on the table right away and state the over-all conclusions to which I have come about psychotherapy.

Firstly, if we are to search for a paradigm for our work, we should look to that of friendship rather than the application of scientific theory.

Secondly, the commonplace attitudes which are relevant to healing lie in the direction of warmth rather than coldness, trust rather than cynicism, closeness rather than distance, encouragement rather than discouragement, spontaneity rather than calculation. This is not to say that the therapist should not, in his efforts to heal, manifest at times attitudes designed to distance and discourage, and might even resort to harsh and devastating criticism, but that such approaches to the other will not be in the ascendant. Let me here risk a word that may seem naïve in this context: the wise man who seeks to heal will, in his dealings with the troubled person, reveal qualities that we normally associate with the word 'good'. And this thought brings problems.

It is not considered unusual for a parent to have a loving attitude towards his child. Similarly, a friend may care for another, or someone may go to help an injured or sick person, without attracting comment. But if a man were to set himself up and say, 'This is the kind of thing I do. I love my children, I show concern for my friends, I am ready to go to the aid of the sick and injured', we may accuse him of arrogance. It is as if he were saying, 'I thank thee, Lord, that I am not as other men: I am loving, kind and considerate.'

What then of the psychotherapist? A psychotherapist is someone who sets himself up as one who helps others, who publicly announces that he has the necessary qualities. It is true that the saintliness of his position is modified by the fact that he does this for money, but even so he implicitly asserts that he has within him the capacity to help. How are we to think of this assertion? If we are to say, 'He helps by means of a learned technique', then there is no problem. But if we believe that the ability to bring relief to those in anguish depends in no small part on the possession of attributes such as wisdom, lovingness, patience, honesty, etc., then the therapist appears to be in an embarrassing situation. He seems to be saying, 'I have set myself up as a therapist because I have the virtues required of such work.'

I am not alone in openly stating that the therapist's love for his patient often plays a significant part in healing and may even be the crucial factor.[1] How do those – and they are many – who *implicitly* believe in the importance of their caring deal with the charge of arrogance to which they are vulnerable? Primarily, I believe, by evasiveness. They say, 'We all of us, naturally, care for our patients.* This can be taken for granted. It is the baseline of our work, from which the important part emerges, the part we talk about, namely, our technique.' But this statement submerges the truth that non-technical qualities are *central* to healing. And a danger has appeared: that therapist and student may become so preoccupied with technique that their capacity to recognize, and even manifest, human qualities is diminished.

In writing this book, having the set of suppositions about psychotherapy that I have just outlined, I am in a difficult position. How can I describe my work without blushing? How can I avoid giving the impression that I believe my love for my patients to be of sufficient degree to justify writing about it?

But this seemingly presumptuous claim is not as immoderate as might appear. If I say to a colleague (to put it somewhat naïvely), 'I help people by wisdom and love, whereas you rely on technique', it might be taken to imply that I believe I have a greater capacity for loving than he, but I do not think that I am necessarily making such a claim. What I say could have two different meanings. Firstly, 'We both help by wisdom and love but you fail to recognize or acknowledge this fact.' Alternatively, I am saying, 'I know I am not a wiser or more loving person than you but at least I don't wreck such capacity as I have for revealing such virtues by adhering to a theory which neglects their value and even discourages their manifestation.'

Although I believe this claim is not, in fact, arrogant, I have some

* Although the term 'patient' has connotations which make it unsatisfactory in the context of psychotherapy, I use it in this book as I can think of no better substitute.

sympathy with those who view it with suspicion. The temptation to bask in the idea that one is more virtuous than one's fellows is almost irresistible; and patients can all too readily idealize the therapist and tempt him into the belief that he is an uncommonly wise and loving human being. (The virtues which a therapist may care to overvalue in himself are varied; although lovingness is perhaps the commonest, there are of course, others: sensitivity, intelligence, toughness, shrewdness, etc.)

The point I wish to make is not that the therapist who attributes virtues to himself is necessarily under an illusion, but that human pride is such that it is difficult for a practitioner to proclaim that these qualities are important in his field of work. Everything that we have learned about modesty, all our opposition to pride and pomposity, causes us to shrink from such statements. Yet if we are to pursue the truth (as Freud himself advised us to do) we cannot evade the problems which arise from a consideration of the significance of human qualities in healing.

The two questions which first come to my mind are: firstly, how do we distinguish between a personal and a technical response? Can personal responses be studied in the way that technical ones can without destroying what we seek to understand?

Secondly, might it be better to leave the personal features to look after themselves and focus on that which we *can* talk about, namely technique? Is it not possible that the moments in therapy of supreme significance are elusive and contain a quality which cannot be pinned down any more than a poem or a sonnet be satisfactorily dissected?

The factors which make it difficult to approach these questions intelligently are not restricted to those concerning pride and modesty; there is also the matter of rigour. To the extent that we regard psychotherapy as a serious pursuit we will wish to select, train, practise, and research with rigour. But on what kind of basis do we pursue rigour? In this respect psychotherapy is in a peculiar position. If I am a clergyman I would not – as yet – be required to produce statistics or perform experimental work, but I would be expected to know my Bible. If I am a doctor I will have been to medical school and learnt the traditional scientific approach to the functioning of the body. But if I wish to practise psychotherapy it is not at all clear what I should do to best equip myself for this purpose. Even those who pursue the most taxing course available –

a Freudian or Jungian training – are taunted by Behaviourists for their lack of 'scientific rigour', by psychiatrists for their ignorance of applied neurophysiology, by philosophers for their adherence to a nineteenth-century model of the mind, by sociologists for their preoccupation with the individual psyche . . .

As an example of this kind of dilemma I would like to refer to an interesting book written a few years ago by Richard Chessick entitled *Why Psychotherapists Fail*.[2] I will start by – gladly – repeating two quotations from eminent psychoanalysts which strongly reflect my own beliefs and of which Chessick clearly approves:

It seems to me that what is more important . . . is not so much what the analyst says as what he is. It is precisely what he is in the depths of himself – his real availability, his receptivity and his authentic acceptance of what the other is – which gives value, pungency and effectiveness to what he says . . . The communication from one unconscious to another which becomes established in the transference relationship between therapist and patient permits the latter to perceive the profound benevolent attitude of the physician. (S. Nacht, 'Reflections on the Evolution of Psychoanalytic Knowledge', *I.J.P.A.* (1969), 50, 597)

How to teach patience and devotion, tact and timing, decency and tolerance, empathy and intuition, modesty and respect in the face of supporting loyalty and keeping distance, carefulness and courage, honesty and frankness? (Martin Grotjahn, 'Problems and Techniques of Supervision', *Psychiatry* (1955), 18, 9)

Chessick's response to this challenge is interesting. He does not, as would Nacht and Grotjahn, advocate a traditional Freudian training but aims at something wider. Certainly it does not lack rigour. He proposes a curriculum 'based on an eight-hour day, six-day week and four-year duration'. He includes 'a *minimum* reading list in philosophy that ought to be required in the training of every psychotherapist' (Chessick's italics). The formidable list of forty-nine books contains such difficult works as Kant's *Critique of Pure Reason* and is eclectic in nature.

I have much sympathy with Chessick's aims. The endeavour to broaden one's mind with the writings of the great philosophers is surely to be praised and can have a modifying effect on the narrow vision of those who unthinkingly accept the prevailing world view of our time or confine themselves to the theories of one psycho-therapeutic school. Indeed, if he had worded his formula somewhat differently – if he had been content to suggest that such books can be useful to the potential psychotherapist – he would have my support. But his insistence on the necessity of this programme for *all* students suggests an exaggerated view of the relevance of intellectual distinction to the capacity to help others, a fantasy of producing an élite (a race of Plato's philosopher-kings), and a determination to be rigorous *at all costs*. It is not as easy as that. Intellectual sophistication is, alas, no guarantee of the kind of qualities for which Nacht and Grotjahn are looking. Indeed, bookishness can often stand in the way.

Our path lies, I believe, between two extremes. On the one hand is the belief that no teaching is necessary to the practice of psychotherapy; anyone can do it, and therefore no one need bother to learn. On the other hand – and this is the dominant view and one that is characteristic of our insecure culture – no one should be permitted to engage in psychotherapy unless he can show evidence of rigorous training in *some* sort of technique. I am personally convinced that, in view of the prevailing philosophy of our time, the chief danger lies in the second view: we have lost touch with the elemental factors involved in help and we put our faith in the compartmentalized knowledge of the 'specialist'.

The simple notion of 'help' readily evokes in us the suspicion of a well-meaning but naïve, undisciplined, and sentimental approach to the other. Although we may be justified in viewing apparent simplicity with circumspection, we should, I believe, be equally careful in our assessment of operations which show the outward manifestations of rigour. How, for instance, does one listen with rigour? It might seem, at first sight, that a tape-recorder could do the job better than us or, failing electronic aids, we should, in motionless silence, hang upon every word. Yet, on the contrary, I believe that a person may often hear another best – may draw him out and understand him best – when to an outside observer he appears to be engaged in ordinary conversation. The criteria by which we can measure rigour in psychotherapy are therefore not obvious. In seeking for them I would like to quote from another area of study, F. R. Leavis's last book, *The Living Principle: 'English' as a Discipline of Thought*:

The discipline is not a matter of learning a deduced standard logic or an eclectic true philosophy, but rather of acquiring a delicate readiness of apprehension and a quasi-instinctive flexibility of response, these informed by the intuited 'living principle' – the principle implicit in the interplay between the living language and the creativity of individual genius. My 'interplay', which is manifested *in* the language as the writer uses it, is an intimation that I have in mind my point that a language is more than a 'means of expression': it embodies values, constatations, distinctions, promptings, recognitions of potentiality.[3]

It seems to me that a good psychotherapist brings to his work not only a rigour which is the equivalent of the close attention to the text required of the literary critic but a comprehensive view of life of a kind which permits an enhancement of living in another human being – an attitude which transcends the particular discipline he has chosen to follow. He will stand or fall by his ability to foster a creative advance in another and, although the *circumstances* of his task are unique, his general aim is similar to that of all those who are concerned with personal growth. These two requirements – a focus on another person in a certain situation and a capacity to foster growth – do not always go together. The first may occur without the second – and we have an observer. The second may occur without the first – and we have a helpful person in a non-psychotherapeutic situation. But they will both be present when someone with a healing attitude makes a serious attempt to help another.

If one were to imagine a continuum of the appropriate predominance of 'scientific' or 'ordinary' perception in various areas of living then psychotherapy would come somewhere in the middle, and it is to this fact that we must attribute the main cause of its present state of confusion. It is less a science than a craft, but it is a craft the aptitude for which derives more from a general experience of living than is usually supposed. In this respect it has much in common with teaching and I would like to make a comparison between the kind of help offered to a child by the two disciplines.

In our society the child is taught at first by ordinary people: his parents. After a certain age, however, experts begin to play an important part in his education. Although parents may have vested interests in their children which interfere with their capacity to foster growth, it is, on the whole, commonly accepted that they are the best people to bring up their offspring. There is sound sense in this notion. The love, devotion, dedication, and sacrifice required over the years to enable a child to flourish is not often to be found outside a family (a fact which is neglected by those writers who have in recent years made a savage attack on the family, basing their criticism on studies of failure).

In certain ways and under certain conditions the task of bringing up a child is too heavy upon the parents, particularly in these days when the extended family has largely disappeared and the technicalities of living and working have become so complicated; and therefore additional help is required. If our society were one in which a sense of community was dominant – instead of one committed, as Philip Slater puts it, to the 'pursuit of loneliness'[4] – then help would be more readily available than it is at present. As things stand, however, help is given in a highly organized system of institutions: by education, health, and the social services. If all appears well for the child then society leaves him alone except for the requirement that he attend school, a place where it is assumed he will be provided with a kind of help which is beyond the capacities of the parents. If, on the other hand, things go wrong, then a doctor or a social worker will be called in for advice.

Whether the required help is of a technical nature or not is clearly an important matter in considering what resources in society can be tapped. Certain factors in the fields of both education and medico-social welfare are undoubtedly specialized, e.g. a family is unlikely to be able to provide the know-how or facilities to teach advanced chemistry or remove an inflamed appendix. But when one comes to consider the sort of help a child may require which is not technical (or, at least, not so obviously and overwhelmingly technical), we are then faced with the more ordinary kinds of help – that of enabling a child to grow in the way that is best for him – which depend less on specialized training than on interest, patience, a knowledge of children, and, not least, a sufficiency of time. The aim is focused upon the child as a whole and the object is to enable him to fulfil his potentiality in whatever way is best for him personally, given the sort of society he will have to face as an adult. If this endeavour is directed towards a child considered to be healthy it is called education (in the sense of the term as used, for instance, by Froebel); if towards a child deemed to be sick or maladjusted it is called psychotherapy (or a similar name to refer to some form of counselling). It would appear therefore that education and psychotherapy are terms used to refer to a basically similar ideal; that of promoting an undistorted growth of the child's self. Some methods of approach used by teacher and therapist will not be common to both: a therapist may feel somewhat inadequate if faced with a room full of children all expecting to be taught a certain subject, and a teacher may not feel too happy about the way to respond to a 6-year-old's sexual fantasies. Whether or not the ability to deal well with each of these situations should be called a technical one is debatable, for many people would, I think, consider it to depend on one's *experience* of children in each kind of situation. The point I wish to make here is that in both situtations the capacity to help is based, in no small part, on the kind of understanding which is open to people who are neither teachers nor therapists, but who have somehow acquired the interest in and knowledge of what makes us tick, and an intuitive sense of how to get the best out of us, whether we want to learn how to swim or to overcome an anxiety about swimming.

In his book *Education for Liberation*, Adam Curle writes, in a chapter entitled 'A Possible Future':

Certainly everything will depend upon the quality of the teachers. It always has done, of course, but now that education is so vast an industry and the standards of teaching so various, many students learn more from good books than from poor teachers. For the sort of education which I envisage, however, supremely good teachers are indispensable. They must be able to sense the latent capacities, the potential lines of development, the inner blockages and confusions, of every child. They must appreciate many kinds of growth, including those which the system today ignores or despises, and recognise that they may represent perfection for a given individual. Finally, they must know what to teach and how to do so in order to fulfil the potentialities of their student's growth.

A first step towards obtaining teachers who can act in this way would be to disestablish the teaching profession (indeed all professions, as we shall see, but teaching first of all). There would be no profession of teachers, no group of young men and women who have made the choice for good reasons or bad to be pedagogues rather than technicians or doctors or advertising agents, or who indeed had no choice about it at all. The teachers of tomorrow would be chosen in mature years (how old this might be varies from person to person) by a commission skilled in identifying wisdom, patience, sincerity, warmth, and inner coherence. It matters little how such a person has spent most of his or her life – as a stone mason, computer expert, physician, cook, waitress, farmer or poet.[5]

Curle's requirements for the selection of teachers are similar to the ones I myself would advocate in the case of those wishing to practise psychotherapy, although I think he overlooks the difficulty

– if not impossibility – of finding 'a commission skilled in identifying wisdom'.

I do not think that the current reliance on technique is merely a defensive manoeuvre to avoid facing the problem of wisdom – although a good case could be made for thinking that this emphasis is, in fact, a major distortion of contemporary culture. But, whatever the origin of this emphasis, our pressing concern is its consequence in psychotherapy today. What I wish to pursue in this book is the possibility of describing a psychotherapy which makes wise dealing its central feature rather than an attribute which has slipped in through the back door.

We now come to another paradox. If, in order to help another, I need wisdom, is there an in-built inequality between myself and my patient? Is it a case of the wise leading the un-wise? And, if I present myself to him in this way, may I not increase his sense of inferiority and provoke his envy? The formal situation in which one person tries to help another has inherent problems for both parties irrespective of the nature of the disability for which help is sought, and one of the most difficult and important of these problems is the question of equality. Let me give an example.

A young man recently started therapy with me. One day he observed that I appeared to be feeling low. I acknowledged that this was indeed the case and told him, as simply as I could, the reason for my state of mind. A week later we started to discuss his extreme competitiveness, the degree to which it pervaded his relationships, the subtle ways in which he concealed its activity. He said: 'Sometimes I can feel one up on another person by being more ill than him, sometimes less ill. It depends on circumstances'. I replied, 'When you are with me it seems to be the latter. You are very composed. My fantasy is that if one of us reveals a messyness it will be me.' He then referred to my having admitted I felt low a week earlier. 'I was glad you made that admission', he said, 'You may have thought that I was concerned about you, but I think it was more that I wanted to bring you down from your professional thing.'

We talked about his dislike of my professional attitude for a while; then I said, 'I think we could go wrong in two ways. On one extreme we would arrive here one day and you would say, "I'm ill, I need help," and I would say, "I'm ill, I need help". And nothing would happen. On the other extreme I would remain hidden and invulnerable behind my professional wall and you would remain feeling one down. We need to work out an acceptable way of being with each other so that, by and large, *I* will try to help *you* but everything else between us is in question.'

In describing this interchange I do not mean to imply that psychotherapy is purely a matter of finding a way of avoiding unnecessary inequality between therapist and patient, but I do believe that it is very difficult to help someone unless this particular problem is faced and, to a degree, overcome, for it is inevitably a central issue to those who seek help because they do not feel 'equal' to their fellow men.

There is a deep distrust of professionalism, albeit often unconscious, in many who seek therapeutic help, and this does not depend only upon the sense of inequality which the situation fosters. Another aspect of the problem was put to me recently by a man who came because he was unhappy, did not know what to do with his life, and wondered whether psychotherapy might help. He had an anguished look about him and he spoke quickly and jerkily. At one point in the interview he expressed his doubts.

'It seems somehow too materialistic. I pay you and you give me your time. Yes, I know you need money, everybody needs money. But it's not – what's the word, I don't know – "spiritual"? We'll go through a lot of talk and you'll tell me things but there will be something missing. Let me say what I want in life (you'll probably think I'm an incurable Romantic and perhaps I am). Sometimes someone smiles at me. I may not know him – or her. Perhaps they don't know anything about me – I might be a criminal, I might be the organizer of all the prostitution in the world – but to them, at that moment, it doesn't matter. And I'll smile back. Without something like that my life's just a sham.'

Whether or not his 'incurable Romanticism' was a fault is a questionable matter. It certainly may have a bearing on his anguish. But the point he makes would find agreement with those who seek – in life and in therapy – something beyond an exchange between people who are functioning primarily on the basis of their role. In a critique of the 'ethnomethodologists' Edmond Ions writes:

As with Garfinkel, a persistent, indeed a universal theme in Goffman's writings is that in their social relations, people are essentially actors, playing roles and putting on performances. The theatrical metaphor is sometimes replaced by a sporting one, where 'players', 'games' and 'teams' replace 'actors'. Common to both Garfinkel and Goffman is a view of human interaction as essentially a performance, assumed or enlisted by the individual in order to 'score' off opponents, real, potential, or imagined. What is absent is any discussion of such elements of human interaction as compassion, sympathy, charity, or love – to name only a few. A child reared on an exclusive diet of Goffman's writings would have no acquaintance with anything that could be termed a moral universe. Life would consist of actors acting out self-assumed roles, alternating with gamesters permanently taking on, or putting down, opponents by means of various stratagems. A person would be no more than a performance, or a set of performances. There would be no further mysteries to the self – that is to say, none that could not be abstracted or deduced from outward and visible performances.

Goffman and Garfinkel belong essentially to the behavioural school of overt performances. Their drastic and diminishing view of personality seems to me dangerously incomplete. One can concede Goffman's social observations on 'the calculative, gameslike aspects of mutual dealings' without conceding that his is in any sense a complete or even an adequate account of human interaction. A clue to that inadequacy is provided by the titles to three of Goffman's books: 'Where the Action is'; 'Strategic Interaction'; and 'Interaction Ritual'. Throughout, the discussion centres on observed 'behavioural' exchanges. Action is being, and being is action. Inaction provides no clues to the individual or to self. A person is a being engaged in a game, or a series of games – no less and no more.

It is here that the affinity with earlier, cruder forms of role theory and behaviourism is much closer than Goffman's apologists recognise.[6]

The danger which Ions identifies extends, increasingly, into the field of psychotherapy. The more the therapist and patient are conceived in terms of actors or performers the more the essence of a fruitful engagement is lost. What can sometimes be of most use to a patient (whether child or adult) is precisely the absence of a response that is designed to be therapeutic or could be formulated in words as a piece of therapeutic work. Perhaps such a reaction may make up for a deprivation in ordinary responses in earlier life, but it is unlikely to achieve this if it is a deliberate attempt to perform in this way. And I do not wish to suggest that a spontaneous reaction should be a paradigm for therapeutic action any more than the considered reflective responses that occur when the therapist is preoccupied with his role and may organize his behaviour to this end and describe it as technique.

Because psychotherapy is at present so ill defined and so beset with controversy about its nature (to some aspects of which I have already called attention) I shall, in this book, approach it from different angles and try to throw light on some of the reasons for its present state of disarray. One of the many causes of trouble is the fact that, although our society is addicted to the formation of distinctions, there is no clarity in those which are often made between psychotherapy and related forms of helping people. Many people assume a progression from simple to specialized help – from 'befriending' to 'counselling' to 'psychotherapy' and then on to 'psychoanalysis' – yet find great difficulty in formulating the nature of the differences. I believe these distinctions are artificial and misleading and depend, in no small degree, on our craving for status. It is therefore necessary to say that, while there is a difference in the *intensity* of need of certain individuals and of the help offered to them, there is not necessarily any basic difference in the *nature* of the transaction. I shall, in what follows, use the term 'psychotherapy' to include all formal encounters in which one person aims to help the being of another in a way that does not primarily depend on the use of physical techniques, conversion to dogma, or deception.

I am writing about psychotherapy and not about philosophy, and I shall not dwell on the latter; nor shall I pursue the Marxist view that our social theories derive from political motives. There are many works which undermine the positivism on which the day-to-day practice, discussion, and documentation of psychotherapy, psychiatry, and social science relies. I shall quote only one.

F. A. Hayek ended his Nobel Memorial Lecture with the following words, which, although derived from his work in economics and philosophy, apply with even greater force to psychotherapy:

If man is not to do more harm than good in his efforts to improve the social order, he will have to learn that in this, as in all other fields where essential complexity of an organised kind prevails, he cannot acquire the full knowledge which would make mastery of the events possible. He will therefore have to use what knowledge he can achieve, not to shape the results as the craftsman shapes his handiwork, but rather to cultivate a growth by providing the appropriate environment, in the manner in which the gardener does this for his plants. There is danger in the exuberant feeling of ever growing power which the advance of the physical sciences has engendered and which tempts man to try, 'dizzy with success', to use a characteristic phrase of early communism, to subject not only our natural but also our human environment to the control of a human will. The recognition of the insuperable limits to his knowledge ought indeed to teach the student of society a lesson in humility which should guard him against becoming an accomplice in men's fatal striving to control society – a striving which makes him not only a tyrant over his fellows, but which may well make him the destroyer of a civilisation which no brain has designed but which has grown from the free efforts of millions of individuals.

The analogy with gardening is apt. But if I were to write a book about gardening I could assume, without drawing attention to the fact, that sun, moisture, earth, and seeds are of ultimate importance in the growth of plants, and I would have a body of scientific know-ledge (biology) to support me in the unlikely case of my assumption meeting a challenge. I would therefore write about the techniques of gardening. But in writing about psychotherapy the position is quite different. We have only hazy notions about the forces that enable *people* to grow, or even about what we mean by growth in the human context. We cannot therefore speak of a technique of psychotherapy without making unwarranted assumptions about matters which are in need of greater understanding.

Because I have been so influenced by Freud I would like, at this point, to state briefly my position in regard to Freudian theory.

There is at present no satisfactory definition of psychotherapy. The fact that schools of thought so drastically in opposition to each other as the 'psychodynamic' and 'behaviouristic' gather together in an effort to prescribe acceptable credentials for the practice of 'psychotherapy' is evidence of this. Almost everything I have learned in life and therapy leads me to favour the 'dynamic' school if by this remarkably inappropriate term one refers to a focus on the experiential, intuitive, empathic, receptive, historical approach which characterizes the attitude of those who march under this banner. I will go further and say that, in my view, the contribution of the Freudian school to what I understand by the term psycho-therapy is by far the richest source available to anyone who wishes to work in this field.

Robert Heilbroner explains 'the reason for the magnetism that Marx exerts' as follows:

It is that Marx had the luck, combined of course with the genius, to be the first to discover a whole mode of inquiry that would forever after belong to him. This was done previously only once, when Plato 'discovered' the mode of Philosophical inquiry.

To be sure, there had been philosophical explorations before Plato, bold forays by brilliant men, above all the luminous figure of Socrates. But if Plato was not the first to ask philosophical questions, he was the first to systematize the method of posing and considering these questions, so that later thinkers, no matter how great or original, found themselves pursuing a task whose nature was still essentially that articulated by Plato. That is why, in a sense all of philosophy is a commentary on Plato's work, even when it goes far beyond Plato or arrives at conclusions that are completely at variance with his own. So it is with Marx.

Pursuing the question of Marx's hold over us, Heilbroner continues

. . . It is certainly not because he is infallible. It is because he is un-avoidable, at least for anyone who begins to ask questions, not about society but about the nature of our thinking about society. Sooner or later, all such inquiries bring one to confront Marx's thought, and then one is compelled to adopt, confute, expand, escape from, or come to terms with the person who has defined the very task of critical social inquiry itself.[7]

What Heilbroner affirms about Plato and Marx is, I believe, true of Freud. He also was the first to 'discover a whole mode of inquiry that would forever after belong to him', and a psychotherapist can no more ignore this contribution than a historian can ignore that of Marx. Nevertheless, we can be philosophers without being Platonists and historians without being Marxists – and so we can be psychotherapists without being Freudians.

Although Freud constructed an impressive intellectual edifice to account for his findings we would be well advised, I think, to make a distinction between the practical and theoretical aspects of his work, for Freud the scientist was called upon to deal in an *ad hoc* manner with real people who sought his help. Leaving aside for the moment the scientific principles which he considered to inform his approach, let us look at what he actually did with people. He invited them into his study and listened carefully and seriously to what they had to say about their predicament. He believed, like Plato, in facing reality and in self-discipline, and he therefore encouraged his patients to take responsibility for their problems and to pursue the truth about themselves no matter how difficult and devious the path. He gave them time, free from the pressure of their normal daily life, in order to do this. Finally, sceptic that he was, he took little for granted and always looked beneath the surface of things. We may, in some ways, quibble with this approach to those in anguish, but it is not a bad recipe. It is a product of common sense, and is founded upon an ancient and well-tried philosophy of living, one calculated to foster stoical qualities in both helper and helped. In simple terms, Freud's achievement was to enable two people to meet each other in order that they may, free from the dogma of religion and illusion of magic, talk about the problem of one of them. This, to my mind, is psychotherapy.

But, being a genius, Freud did more than this. Using whatever sources were at his disposal, including observations in the therapeutic setting, he made formulations about human behaviour which carry such conviction that many of them have not only entered into our intellectual heritage but have become accepted as common knowledge.

This was an act of immense courage, achieved in loneliness.* But even Freud was not able to say (what I believe is nearest the truth) that it was he, Freud, who gave the help, using himself, the totality of his experience. What he did say was: 'It is by science that I help you'. This was his only outside support, his only concession, but it has cost us dear in the end. One wonders how psychotherapy might have developed had Freud not regarded himself as an agent of medical science. Unfortunately, we are now able to hide behind Freud, and to say, as it were: 'It is not I who helps you, but Freud.' In doing so we are saved from the accusation of arrogance (for who am I to set myself up as helper?); but we also avoid full responsibility for what we do. The charge of arrogance is, indeed, one to be taken seriously but I believe we can escape it if we have the humility to recognize that when healing occurs we can only take a limited amount of the credit: not only do the will of the patient and the facilitating situation of therapy play a significant part but there are always healing factors of which we know little or nothing, and (since life is enigmatic) can never hope to know. Our task, in relation to Freud, is to be able to utilize those of his insights and recommendations which make sense to us today without feeling obliged to become converts to his systematization of healing.

A few weeks after an earlier book of mine was published, I received a long and closely argued letter of criticism by a man who

---

* Although Freud's courage is not, to my mind, in doubt, the degree of his intellectual isolation and the empirical sources of his theories have been forcibly challenged by Frank Sulloway in his book *Freud, Biologist of the Mind*, Burnett Books, 1979.

was unknown to me. The critique, by George Craig, included this statement: 'No one has a serene overview of human experience, since to be human is, *inter alia*, to be unable to step outside the limitedness which is our condition. Since that is the case there can be no unchallengable expert – or expertise – in human relations.'

It is difficult to know how we can fruitfully delineate an area of endeavour to be called 'psychotherapy'. But of one thing I am sure. We should not make the mistake of allowing a rationally ordered approach towards sickness and healing (or education and morality) to usurp the wisdom which draws its conclusions from data that are complex beyond our understanding. One of the reasons for doing this is our pervasive tendency to disparage the ordinary and worship the special. It is to this mistaken attitude of mind that I now turn.

References

1. Halmos, P. (1965), *The Faith of the Counsellors*, Constable, London.
2. Chessick, R. (1971), *Why Psychotherapists Fail*, Science House, New York.
3. Leavis, F. R. (1975), *The Living Principle: 'English' as a Discipline of Thought*, Chatto and Windus, London, p. 49.
4. Slater, P. (1971), *The Pursuit of Loneliness*, Allen Lane, London.
5. Curle, A. (1973), *Education for Liberation*, Tavistock, London, p. 34.
6. Ions, E. (1978), *Against Behaviourism*, Blackwell, Oxford.
7. Heilbroner, R. (1978), *New York Review of Books*, xxv, no. ii (29 June), 33.

2. The Ordinary and the Special

Humble in a dress that would feed a thousand Indians for a
month, making a variation of that speech which goes: I
wanna thank all them little people without whom there
would be no big people like me. – Stanley Reynolds, writing
in the *Guardian*, on the awards of the American Academy
of Motion Pictures

One day I was discussing with a man his feeling of being special.
'Why are you special?' I asked.

'Because I'm a Jew.'

'Then you feel special as opposed to me since I am not a Jew?'

'Oh, no. You are special too. Because you are a psychoanalyst.'

Instead of making an interpretation I found myself exclaiming:
'But don't you see we are just two ordinary people? We are *not*
special!'

At around the same time in my career I was seeing a very sick
young woman who suffered from anorexia nervosa. For a year or
more she had always been dressed in black and was preoccupied
with suicide. I felt that she taunted me with the threat of suicide and
played on my anxiety. My difficulties were increased by the fact that
she was unwilling to tell me her address (she lived on her own). I
came to an 'agreement' with her that she was entirely responsible
for her life and an 'agreement' with myself that, in so far as I could, I
would not worry about the possibility of suicide.

At the end of one particular session she said good-bye with a
peculiar emphasis. Her tone of voice had an air of finality about it. I
did nothing except to respond with my usual 'good-bye'. She then
went home and killed herself.

It is of course easy to be wise after the event and no event
promotes such a tendency to have regrets than suicide. Perhaps it
was not possible for me to have helped this woman by any measures, but I now believe that anything I might have done or said
would have been preferable to the action I took. It would have been
better to hug her, or hit her. . . . And I think my response was
wrong because it was so totally lacking in spontaneity. Not only did
I behave with professional formality but I acted rigidly in accordance with a planned programme of my own making.

The two experiences I have described, although very different at first sight, have something in common: they are concerned with the conflict between ordinary and special behaviour. They both played a part in my gradual recognition that an ordinary response to people is of far greater importance than I had been led by my teaching to believe.

To emphasize the importance of an unspecialized approach can easily lead one into trouble over the question of 'common sense'. The common-sense man – the man-in-the-street – may react simply and straightforwardly to a person in trouble, and the result may be beneficial. But, on the other hand, his 'common sense' will be a product of the society in which he lives, and his response may well be influenced by the specialists of that society in a way that leads him to depart from a simple and straightforward action. Indeed he may have learned to think of a deeply disturbed person as a 'nut-case' for whom the best place is a mental hospital; and, acting on the basis of this belief, his responses could be inhibited and even inhuman. In using terms such as ordinary, simple, straightforward, or unspecialized, I therefore imply an attitude that does not necess-arily conform to the norms of the society in question. Indeed, such an attitude may, by the standards of the society, be deemed extra-ordinary, freakish, or even immoral. In Hitler's Germany it was not considered ordinary to befriend a Jew.

The psychotherapist who tries to be natural with his patient needs therefore to free himself, as far as possible, not only from the sense of distance which his professional training may have given him but from the prejudices of the common sense of his culture. One may say that the man who can do this would necessarily *be* rather special, in the sense of 'unusual'. But to put it this way merely exemplifies the paradox of words; it is rather like saying that the most typical member of a species is untypical because he is in a unique position.

The dilemma over ordinariness was one with which Kierkegaard was painfully familiar and which he often illuminated brilliantly. For example, in *Fear and Trembling* he describes his ideal: the 'Knight of Faith', who appears at first sight to be a very ordinary man:

Here he is. Acquaintance made, I am introduced to him. The moment I set eyes on him I instantly push him from me, I myself leap backwards, I clasp my hands and say half aloud, 'Good Lord, is this the man? Is it really he? Why, he looks like a tax-collector.' However, it is the man after all. I draw closer to him, watching his least movements to see whether there might not be visible a little heterogenous fractional telegraphic message from the infinite, a glance, a look, a gesture, a note of sadness, a smile, which betrayed the infinite in its heterogeneity with the finite. No! He is solid through and through. His tread? It is vigorous, belong entirely to finiteness; no smartly dressed townsman who walks out to Fresberg on a Sunday afternoon treads the ground more firmly, he belongs entirely to the world, no Philistine more so.

But this simplicity is deceptive:

And yet, and yet – actually I could become furious over it, for envy if for no other reason – this man has made and every instant is making the movements of infinity. With infinite resignation he has drained the cup of life's profound sadness, he knows the bliss of the infinite, he senses the pain of renouncing everything, the dearest things he possesses in the world, and yet finiteness tastes to him just as good as to one who never knew anything higher, for his continuence in the finite did not bear a trace of the cowed and fearful spirit produced by the process of training; and yet he has this sense of security in enjoying it, as though the finite life were the surest thing of all. And yet, and yet the whole earthly form he exhibits is a new creation by virtue of the absurd. He resigned everything infinitely, and then he grasped everything again by virtue of the absurd.[1]

Kierkegaard conveys to us the enormous difficulty – the well-nigh impossibility – of purposefully and creatively renouncing the extraordinary as our goal. And when he speaks of envy of the men who can do it, the thought has peculiar pathos in view of his own inability to be ordinary in everyday life. The predicament he describes is very similar to his actual experience with Regine Olsen, with whom, because of the nature of his temperament, he could only engage at a distance:

Suppose I got married to her. What then? In the course of half a year, in less time than that, she would have torn herself apart. There is – and this is both the good and the bad about me – something ghostly about me, something which accounts for the fact that no one can put up with me who has to see me day by day and thus have a real relation to me . . .[2]

Moreover, at various places in his writings, Kierkegaard gives us ample and moving evidence of his plight in life:

My sorrow is my castle, built like an eagle's nest upon the peak of a mountain lost in the clouds. No one can take it by storm. From this abode I dart down into the world of reality to seize my prey; but I do not remain there. I bear my quarry aloft to my stronghold. My booty is a picture I weave into the tapestries of my palace. There I live as one dead.[3]

It is ironic that the two thinkers – Kierkegaard and Heidegger – who were most influential in philosophy's concern with being-in-the-world were both so contemptuous of the everyday existence of the common man. The sad paradox is that Existentialism is concerned with the idea that reflective thought deprives us of authentic living, yet continues the idealization of the thinker.

There are reasons to believe that our denigration of the ordinary is a product of 'civilization'. Stanley Diamond writes:

The search for the primitive is the attempt to define a primary human potential. Without such a model (or, since we are dealing with men and not things, without such a vision), it becomes increasingly difficult to evaluate or understand our contemporary pathology and possibilities. For instance, without an anthropology bent on rediscovering the nature of human nature, the science of medicine may survive, but the art of healing will wither away. For healing flows from insight into primary, 'pre-civilized' human processes; it presumes a knowledge of the primitive, a sense of the minimally human, a sense of what is essential to being human.

To the primitive acting within the society, the major elements interpenetrate in a circular, self-reinforcing manner: all aspects of behaviour converge in a system that strives toward maximum equilibrium. We, of course, can and do analyse out the component parts of the system; we, as outsiders, can demonstrate that changes in technology, in the mode of making a living or in land tenure introduced by Europeans, shatter the joint family structure, and with it, eventually, ancestor worship; civilization is compelled to dissect the corpses it creates. But the primitive moves within this system as an integrated person. His society is neither compartmentalized nor fragmented, and none of its parts is in fatal conflict with the others. Thus he does not perceive himself as divided into *homo economicus*, *homo religiosus*, *homo politicus* and so forth. For example, the Yir-Yiront, an Australian people, make no linguistic distinction between work and play. The primitive stands at the centre of a synthetic, holistic universe of concrete activities, disinterested in the causal nexus between them, for only consistent crises stimulate interest in the causal analysis of society. It is the pathological disharmony of social parts that compels us minutely to isolate one from another, and inquire into their reciprocal effects.

This personalism is the most historically significant feature of primitive life and extends from the family outward to the society at large and ultimately to nature itself. It seems to underlie all other distinctive qualities of primitive thought and behaviour. Primitive people live in a personal corporate world, a world that tends to be a 'thou' to the subjective 'I' rather than an 'it' impinging upon an objectively separate and divided self. Consciousness, for the primitive, is the most common condition in the universe, a perception that is also found, in more civilized and abstract forms, in the work of Whitehead, Haldane and Teilhard de Chardin.[4]

To what extent we can rid ourselves, in this society, of our need to be specialists – to what extent it is psychologically feasible and socially practical – I do not know, but I believe it should be our aim. Our culture is not the only one which has had to face the problems of specialization (the primitive's simplicity must not be idealized) but we have reached a threshold which makes life almost intolerable for many.

The psychotherapist, then, is not alone in facing this dilemma. But how can he best face it? How can he rid himself of those cultural assumptions that are antagonistic to his work? I am reminded of one of the parables of Chuang-tzu:

Ch'ing, the chief carpenter, was carving wood into a stand for hanging musical instruments. When finished, the work appeared to those who saw it as though of supernatural execution. And the prince of Lu asked him, saying, 'What mystery is there in your art?'

'No mystery, your Highness,' replied Ch'ing, 'and yet there is something. When I am about to make such a stand, I guard against any diminution of my vital power. I first reduce my mind to absolute quiescence. Three days in this condition, and I become oblivious of any regard to be gained. Five days, and I become oblivious to any fame to be acquired. Seven days, and I become unconscious of my four limbs, and my physical frame. Then, with no thought of the Court present in my mind, my skill becomes concentrated, and all disturbing elements from without are gone. I enter some mountain forest, I search for a suitable tree. It contains the form required, which is afterwards elaborated. I see the stand in my mind's eye, and then set to work. Otherwise, there is nothing. I bring my own natural capacity into relation with that of the wood. What was suspected to be of supernatural execution in my work was due solely to this.'

. I know I cannot hope to emulate the old man's capacity for concentration. And I doubt if Chuang-tzu would expect me to try (probably he would laugh at me for taking his parable too seriously). But he speaks of the kind of approach to psychotherapy towards which I believe we should aim. It is not the concentration of conscious effort to perfect a technique or adhere to a theory, but the concentration that appears naturally when one person is interested in another's being. Of the correctness of this approach I have no doubt. How, in our present society, in our professional milieu, with our own practical and narcissistic needs, and our due respect for the work of those who have stressed the technical approach, can we best reach for it? We need to ask such questions as, 'What does it mean to be natural in the psychotherapeutic session? In what ways do we need to be different from our behaviour in ordinary life? At what point and in what way does this difference interfere with our capacity to help?' But before considering these questions in detail, I would like in this chapter to suggest some of the factors that have led us into the present predicament.

That we have become victims of our technological success, that it intrudes into areas of subtle, personal, and private experience, has become almost a truism. Those who have written about it with insight and passion are too numerous to mention. This book is but one more protest against the way in which such thinking cripples our lives. But technology has not only brought us a distorted idea of human relationships: it has played into the hands of mankind's perennial pursuit of certainty. We seek someone who knows. No one conducts this search with greater desperation than the man who has lost his way and needs a guide. Such a man is all too ready to impute special qualities to a prospective helper. And the psychotherapist, in order to prevent discouragement, is tempted to show that he is different from the ordinary run-of-the-mill person.

As an example of the tendency to idealize the helper I will recount the words of a woman who came to me for her first 'treatment' session. At one point she scrutinized me carefully and then laughed: 'You really are a normal size, aren't you? When I came to you before [a few months ago] I had the impression afterwards that you were abnormally large.' She went on to tell me that after the original (assessment) interview she had a dream in which our meeting took place in a huge and impressive mansion with high ceilings and wonderful architecture (a far remove, I might say, from the reality of my consulting room). It is difficult for a therapist to present himself as ordinary yet convey to the patient that he may be able to help, for he is up against all those factors which lead people to admire and follow the extraordinary man. Where does this tendency come from?

The failure to appreciate the worth of an ordinary human being stems, I think, from the inclination to lose our sense of balance when presented with someone or something which *commands* our attention. We are drawn, like moths to a candle, towards those who are reputed to possess superior qualities, and we will all too readily listen to a voice that is strident rather than wise. Even when a person may not impress us by his charisma he may nevertheless gain our hearing if he is seen as someone unusual – a man of connections or a specialist of some kind. Thus, as the cynic well knows, true value is not to be equated with the estimation of society.

Children learn this early. The child who, rightly or wrongly, feels himself to be overlooked, soon discovers ways of behaving which single him out for special notice, for he finds that both family and society are ready to collude with his attempts, to encourage him to be eminent and win acclaim for which those who reared him can take credit.

The recognition of real achievement, whether in child or adult, is surely right and realistic, and it is unwise to give a child the impression that he need make no effort, that whatever he does, good or bad, strong or feeble, courageous or timid, is equally worthy of regard. But there is a great difference between the simple and sober response to accomplishment and the idealization of success. In the latter case the child is encouraged to shine rather than be, to triumph rather than meet, to be specialized rather than whole, to seek praise rather than create – and to despise the ordinary. This tendency is so widespread – and in my view so harmful – that I would like to pursue further the reasons for its remarkable persistence in society.

Fear is a natural and healthy reaction to danger but one which can all too easily degenerate into unhealthy chronic anxiety. And, in the same way, an alertness to the unusual and a respect for the powerful and thrusting have undoubted survival value, but may well decline into a timid, passive, and lazy acceptance of the line of least resistance. Not only does it require less courage to accept the hypnotizing certainties of those who appear to know or are said to know, but it is, in this subtle and confusing world, intellectually easier. And so (as Freud noted with such profit) we idealize the powerful, those whom we have cause to fear, or from whom, in our vulnerability, we need help. But to the extent that we focus upon the obvious and disturbing we neglect the ordinary; we are unable to see the significance of that which presents itself quietly, with humility or sophistication; we are blinded by the bright light and cannot perceive those things which are revealed in a gentler illumination.

When behaviour is of a kind which is merely fashionable or

superficially arresting – when its effect depends on an ability to perform in a manner calculated to impress a society which lays down certain arbitrary standards of excellence – it is not too difficult to find evidence of idealization. In the case of genius the matter is different. Although it is possible to idealize the St Matthew Passion or the sculptures of Michelangelo, it would be churlish to stress this theoretical possibility rather than to acknowledge their power to stir our imagination. But the fact that, even in such a case, we are not free from the tendency to idealize the extraordinary shows itself in our equation of the man and his work: in the frequent assumption (despite biographical evidence to the contrary) that the superiority of the works is matched by a superiority of their creator. Yet, on the contrary, there is much to suggest that the work of the genius is often a complicated attempt to overcome a failure to be ordinary.

In his book *Creative Malady* Charles Pickering quotes an extract from Proust's *A la recherche du temps perdu*:

'My sole consolation when I went upstairs for the night was that Mama would come in and kiss me after I was in bed. But this goodnight lasted for so short a time: she went down again so soon that the moment in which I heard her climb the stairs, and then caught the sound of her garden dress of blue muslin, from which hung little tassels of plaited straw, rustling along the double-doored corridor, was for me a moment of the keenest sorrow. So much did I love that goodnight that I reached the stage of hoping that it would come as late as possible, so as to prolong the time of respite during which Mama would not yet have appeared. Sometimes when, after kissing me, she opened the door to go, I longed to call her back, to say to her, "Kiss me just once again" . . .'

Pickering makes the following comment on this passage:

Why then did Proust write a masterpiece while I have not? A difference of talent no doubt. Moreover Proust was rich and never had to earn his living. While Proust was able to devote his whole talent to creating his book, I was leading an extremely busy life of practice, teaching, research and public affairs. But there is another great difference. While I was devoted to my mother, as he was to his, and while I had more need of her, since my father died when I was three, my 'Recherche du temps perdu' would not have lingered or indeed referred to any incident when my mother withheld the goodnight kiss. If she did so, I have no memory of it whatsoever.[5]

That Proust's achievement is intimately related to a failure in love is hardly in doubt; but this can be understood in different ways. Pickering appears to suggest that Proust's peculiarity was an excessive love for his mother, whose over-protectiveness he used for the purpose of artistic creativity. I would rather incline to the view that Proust was unable to love his mother as a real person and wrote his masterpiece in an attempt to recreate what he could not have in actuality.

The attitude of the genius to ordinariness is complex. In so far as he has failed to achieve ordinary experience he attempts, by his creative works, to find a way back to the lost wholeness. In so doing he can sometimes bring glimpses of simplicity which are out of our reach most of the time. It is by virtue of his gifts – and his ruthless dedication to their use – rather than his basic experience that he is extraordinary; in most ways he suffers the same joys and sorrows as the rest of us. But in so far as he has rejected the ordinary and focused on the creation of an alternative world his attitude to the former is not unusually one of contempt.

I must not give the impression that I think that enlightenment does not often come as a consequence of giftedness, adventurous risk, endurance, sustained thought, or suffering. It is rather that I wish to convey my belief – which I emphasize here because I think it important to an understanding of the nature of psychotherapy – that a person may achieve as much fullness as we can hope for in this world in the course of a life that does not necessarily give him a special place in society as an outstanding person; that the drive to achieve such a place (whatever gains may or may not result) is all too often a defensive flight from a simple experience which was dearly wished for yet unobtainable; and that ordinary living is not without its own magic, mystery, ecstasy, despair. To put the matter another way: the thesis that I aim to present in this chapter is that the attempt to classify people according to an *over-all* scale of value is misguided and intrinsically impossible.

In the light of this discussion, what, we might ask, does the psychotherapist offer his patient? Does he help him to become an ordinary or a special person? What, in relation to this question, are the needs and wishes of those who ask for help?

Most people who seek psychotherapy have a low evaluation of themselves, although they have tried to overcompensate for this belief: the more disturbed the patient, the lower his self-esteem. In his book *A Home for the Heart* Bruno Bettelheim describes in detail the kind of ambience that is necessary for seriously disturbed people to feel valuable:

Since mental patients feel totally devalued, we can help them regain their sanity only if they can feel from the beginning that the mental hospital is a place that is entirely there for them, that they are all-important, and that there the very best is not too good for them. Then it will be possible to silence the overpowering voice within them, which tells them that they are no good at all.[6]

The first and foremost need of such people is to be accepted, simply, as human beings; in the same way that, one imagines, the first need of a baby is to be accepted as himself. Most of those who come for help are not as sick as the people described by Bettelheim; they have more self-respect and their hunger for validation is not so acute. None the less (at least in my own experience) the need is still paramount and becomes a major concern in therapy. The defence-mechanisms described by Freud are, in the main, designed to conceal this need (although he by no means always formulated them in these terms), and the attention he gave to 'narcissistic' and 'omnipotent' fantasies implies that the reality he urged upon his patients is one based on their ordinary capacities rather than exceptional ability or status. Yet, paradoxically, this was hardly an ethos with which Freud himself appeared to be at ease. He was a person of burning ambition, whose mother expected him to be a great man; whose arrogant confidence in his own viewpoint was his strength; whose opinion of mankind in general and women and children in particular was low. And psychoanalysis has subsequently shown a marked tendency to élitism. Psychoanalysts, as a group, have enormous respect for intellectual distinction; they are drawn, by and large, from the socially and professionally elect and usually command a notable erudition; they aim to achieve a respectable place among scientists; the structure of their institutes is hierarchical; they tend to form cliques; and many believe themselves to be in possession of a method (Freud's 'pure gold') which not only surpasses all others but has little to learn from them. How much of this élitism filters through to the patient in the consulting room? How easy is it, with this background, for the psychoanalyst to feel himself to be an ordinary person? How easy for his patient to present himself as ordinary without a sense of inferiority in the face of such formidable intellectual confidence? And, quite apart from the particular historical context of psychoanalysis, there are many factors which stand in the way of a sense of equality; the therapist has the social status of the professional middle class which the patient does not necessarily possess;* he believes the language used in daily life (i.e. that used by his patient) to be inferior as a means of communication in the psychotherapeutic encounter to the one he uses himself; and he usually considers himself to be able to explore, infinitely more adequately than his patient, what passes between them. Whereas the patient only sees the surface of things the therapist (in his view) is the only one of the two capable of seeing the profundities which lie beneath. It must be clear to the reader that I regard these assumed inequalities open to question.

The extent to which in actual practice patient and analyst fall into the trap of idealization of the therapeutic language is difficult to assess. That good work is undoubtedly done by psychoanalysts in spite of a structured inequality is, I believe, a complex matter, and much can be attributed to the triumph of common sense and other human qualities over unsound traditions and mistaken theoretical assumptions. Practitioners exist whose humility shines out and transcends all theory.

Psychoanalysis has, I believe, strayed away from a correct perception of reality in two different ways (a combination which is remarkably confusing). It is, at the same time, both too prosaic and too imaginative. It is prosaic in its attempts to confine the richness of human experience within an inappropriate scientific idiom; and it is over-imaginative in that it dwells on the almost infinite symbolic meanings of an experience to an extent that detracts from the experience itself. These two paths of departure are forms of specialization: there is an excessive use of (to use Liam Hudson's terms[7]) either convergence or divergence. In our attempts to find a path between these extremes it is important to distinguish two ways in which the word ordinary may be used: the first (and the one that I use throughout this book) denotes the Greek affirmation of wholeness, a conception which neither denies nor overvalues the two frameworks of thought; the second use of the word describes the arid way of life from which these two modes have been extracted. (Unhappily this latter state is all too common: it is a paradox that its frequency derives in part at least from the fact that by failing to value truly ordinary experience, by putting scientific and imagina-

---

* Some of the consequences of the social status of psychoanalysis have been discussed from a Marxist point of view by Robert Castel in *Le Psychoanalysme: l'ordre psychoanalytique et le pouvoir*, François Maspero, 1973.

tive behaviour into special categories, we deprive ourselves of their use except in special circumstances.)

The dangers of the deprivation of the imaginative realm have been perceived, in the field of poetry, in an acute article by Colin Falk. While recognizing that poets needed to emancipate themselves from the 'otherworldliness' of the Symbolists he views with dismay the impoverishment of much contemporary poetry:

If poetry can believe in ordinariness and at the same time in the possibility of its being transcended (whether by mythic or whatever other means) it will be doing a better service to life than it will by making a virtue out of temporary necessity or a world-philosophy out of parochialism . . . If poets will continue to accept ordinariness as the starting-point for their insights rather than lock-stock-and-barrel, as the necessary first word rather than the inescapable last, who can say what salvation of the human state they may not be able to help us towards? The dead weight of what is now ordinariness for most of us may eventually be lifted, the luminous details set free from the mechanised and alienating banality by which they are at present obscured. If this happens, the poetic enterprise will have a lot in common, as it always has done, with the philosophies of human liberation and will remain their 'permanent basis'; the 'alternative reality' we 'gain entry into' will be a better world we have built with our own hands . . . The time has come – we seem to feel – for a reconnection with common sense, not simply as one more swing of the pendulum but as a permanent recognition of where the future of our poetry must lie.[8]

Another source of imaginative sterility is the application of scientific theory to personal reality which, although still a very potent force, has, in the last hundred years, been subjected to a fair amount of criticism. But the critics of scientific method do not usually leave the ordinary man in any better shape than they do the scientist; true vision is considered to be a feat quite beyond both. No discipline of thought has opposed the viewpoint of common sense with greater vigour than academic psychology. In a recent historical survey of his subject, however, Joynson maintains that the 'introspectionism' of the nineteenth century lost favour not only because of the increasing prestige of the natural sciences but because anthropologists were at that time reporting on the widespread and unrealistic tendency of 'primitive' societies to personify inanimate matter, and that these revelations brought all *personal* assessments into disrepute, even those made by people about people or about themselves. This left a clear path open for a movement which culminated in the outright rejection of common sense by Watsonian Behaviourism. But, since the beginning of *gestalt* theory, there has always been a counter-attack, and this is growing in strength. Joynson writes:

There are certain beliefs about human beings which we rarely try to formulate clearly in our daily lives, but which nevertheless seem to be implicit in the way we treat each other, and which come to the fore if we compare ourselves with inanimate beings. We regard ourselves as knowing, feeling and willing creatures, and therefore not as mere bodies, but as mind and body in one. We think we are not wholly determined by factors over which we have no control, but are self-determining and therefore responsible at least in part for our actions and our character. We possess a certain unity and individuality, such that our nature cannot be analysed into elements which lack the quality of the whole. We are aware of moral and aesthetic values, and we believe that we possess a knowledge ourselves which is, in the last resort, inaccessible to others. To the layman, these beliefs – however crudely expressed – are essential to the notion of a person.[9]

Psychoanalysis, in contrast to behaviourism, devotes itself to *subjective* experience and therefore – despite the criticisms to which it is open – lies closer to common sense and therefore is in less danger of removing itself completely from the springs of life. It is, indeed, a huge advance upon the structured inequality of the scientist who seeks to objectify, and a powerful claim has been made for it to be considered, as a branch of hermeneutics (the art or science of interpretation), as a true dialogue between equals.[10] To my mind such a claim must be treated with reservation if the analyst continues to believe that the basis of a fruitful encounter depends upon a privileged access to knowledge provided by his own particular conceptual framework.

I shall now give two simple examples in an attempt to show the degree to which a professional's response depends on his ordinary sensitivity rather than his specialized knowledge.

A teacher at a primary school mentioned to me that a child had said to her: 'Guardian angels watch over me while I'm asleep, don't they?' The teacher found this a difficult question. On what basis could she look for an answer? Her religious beliefs? Her training in the techniques of teaching? Her knowledge of developmental theory? Her experience of children, as a teacher and as a mother?

Her knowledge of this particular child and his home? Or, something that included and transcended all these – something that might be called wisdom? But, whichever the case, the answer was not incidental to the child's schooling; it may have been the most significant thing he 'learned' that day.

The second example is an account of a consultation. A woman whose son suffers from a long-standing psychological illness told me that at one time she consulted a well-known authority on this particular condition. The consultation was traumatic for her. 'He made me feel that it was all my fault. Even after all these years I still feel angry with him.'

Let us assume, for the sake of argument, that the woman is reporting accurately. It would appear that the doctor failed to consider the effect of his criticism in a setting in which the mother was not given sufficient opportunity to understand how she might repair the damage to her son. It also seems likely that his comments were made in a manner which was too judgemental.

In sum I would say that ordinariness is the absence of idealization; it is a state of mind in which everything is given its proper due and appropriate meaning in relation to the whole. Thus all experiences have potential value, although, according to taste and personal history, some will have more interest for each of us than others. When this simple approach to life fails we either make a selection from the available data and accentuate certain items out of all proportion to the rest (in acute form this constitutes fetishism or addiction) or we manufacture an alternative reality in which the whole of life is imbued with a certain quality (dramatization in the case of hysteria, rationality in the case of obsessional neurosis, menace in the case of paranoia). In seriously disturbed people it is not difficult to spot the distortion. But the tenor of living can become twisted in a way which is accepted as normal yet lacks the spontaneity and simplicity of wholeness – a deception which requires continual vigilance to maintain. Much of the work of the psychotherapist lies, I believe, in the unmasking of this deception, a task which he has little chance of performing well unless he is himself relatively free from the idealization of specialized experience.

We therefore must look carefully – and this I propose to do in the next chapter – at the circumstances of a therapeutic meeting with the aim of assessing the degree to which help is a function of the setting itself as opposed to the theoretical presuppositions of the practitioner.

References

1. Kierkegaard, S. (1968), *Fear and Trembling*, trans. Walter Lowrie, Princeton Univ. Press, Princeton, p. 49.
2. Thompson, J. (1974), *Kierkegaard*, Gollancz, London, p. 113.
3. Ibid., p. 128.
4. Diamond, S. (1975), *In Search of the Primitive*, Transaction Books, New Brunswick, p. 495.
5. Pickering, G. (1974), *Creative Malady*, George Allen and Unwin, London, p. 231.
6. Bettelheim, B. (1970), *A Home for the Heart*, Thames and Hudson, London, p. 95.
7. Hudson, L. (1968), *Contrary Imaginations*, Penguin, London.
8. Falk, C. (1974), 'Poetry and Ordinariness', *New Review*, 1, 1.37.
9. Joynson, R. B. (1974), *Psychology and Common Sense*, Routledge and Kegan Paul, London, p. 105.
10. Steele, R. S. (1979), 'Psychoanalysis and Hermeneutics', *Int. Review of Psychoanalysis*, 6, 389.

3. The Situation of Psychotherapy*

Man is all weaknesse, there is no such thing
  As Prince or King:
His arm is short; yet with a sling
  He may do more. – George Herbert, 'Praise'

Let us start with an imaginary person, John Smith, who is in trouble. John is anguished, confused, and in despair. Although he can give some explanations for his unhappy state of mind his condition seems to be out of proportion to any obvious cause. Those around him – relatives, friends, workmates – have tried to help him but he is not very ready to confide in them and they themselves do not feel adequately equipped to deal with someone in this frame of mind. It could be that in another society, one in which people felt more able to be intimate, more ready to turn to others than seeking out an expert of some kind, and more able to expose their weaknesses without fear of ridicule or condemnation, John Smith could find the necessary help from those near to him. But he does not live in such a society. Moreover, because he does not consider himself to be a religious man he hesitates to turn to a priest for succour, and he has little faith that the medicaments of doctors are relevant to his problem. To whom shall he turn? He may seek help from a community (a place to live), a group, or a person. It is with the last of these three possibilities that I am concerned here – although I hope that, because the nature of help transcends specific situations, what I have to say will have some bearing on all three.

Approaching this question from a naïve beginning, it would seem that the person most likely to help is one to whom he could bring his despair without damaging consequences; who would not regard him as silly, unworthy, alien, inferior, or a nuisance, or be overwhelmed by his anguish or demands; who would be able to get close enough to know what he is really like and to feel the genuine interest in him that comes with intimacy; someone ready and able to spend time pursuing the subtleties that foster or obstruct intimacy.

A psychotherapist is, to my thinking, a person who would aim to give this kind of help to John Smith. In order to do so he should be able to behave in certain ways towards him: to show honesty,

* The chapter is developed from an article 'The Nature of Psychotherapy' in Tract No. 23, The Gryphon Press, Sussex.

integrity, rigour, warmth, openness, courage, sensitivity, tolerance, humility, and so on. He would also need to have some experience of trouble: an awareness of what it feels like to be in anguish (both from his own life and from being with others in that state of mind) and of the ways in which people try to avoid awareness of their anguish. This is already a tall order and one which most, if not all, of us will be unable to reach; but there is more. The psychotherapist needs to be in a calm frame of mind – relatively free from distracting anxieties, interruptions, or other preoccupations – so that he can approach the other person with peacefulness and attention; and he must believe that it is right and proper for him to offer himself in this way.

This description of the psychotherapist's attitude does not require the prospective practitioner to learn any scientific theory or religious dogma. He need make no claim to be a Freudian, Jungian, or Christian; have no degree in medicine or psychology, nor have had any formal training in anything whatsoever before embarking on his quest to learn the art of therapy. This is not, of course, to suggest that the great thinkers of the past (or present) have nothing to offer someone who seeks to understand and help his fellows. But what I am searching for at this point, approaching the problem from as simple and logical a position as I can achieve, are the fundamental criteria that need to be met if one person is likely to help another, for this question must come before further questions – however important – of the kind: 'To what extent does possession of Freudian (or Kleinian, or Rogerian, or Behaviouristic, etc.) theory increase the likelihood of helping another?' Our preliminary search for the facilitating circumstances in which healing can help may lead us to an answer to these questions – but that remains to be seen.

Many factors, therefore, are clearly of importance in the outcome of any psychotherapeutic endeavour. These include the following:

1. The social (or professional) set-up in which the two people meet: the therapist's view of the principles surrounding the undertaking.

2. The nature of the two people and the degree of their compatibility.

3. The potentiality for health in the patient.

4. The potentiality for healing – for promoting growth in others – of the therapist.

5. The therapist's particular experience of being with and helping troubled people and the help he himself has received from others in the form of therapy and teaching.

6. The truth of falseness of his theories about the practice of psychotherapy.

In this chapter I wish to focus mainly on the first of these considerations. In order to get a better perspective on this question let us take a further look at the reasons why John Smith may not be able to obtain help from those around him and contrast their position with that of the therapist.

1. He may be a lonely man, alienated from family and society.

2. His relatives may have already taken as much of the burden of his sorrows as they can, or as he feels justified in allowing them to take.

3. There may be such long-standing, complex, and rigid confusions and disharmonies between John and those with whom he lives that an outside view is necessary to understand what is really happening. Indeed, such disharmony may be a contributory, or even the main, cause of his suffering.

4. Because it is shameful, in our society, to admit weakness, there is need of a person who proclaims a different philosophy, to whom someone in trouble may turn without fear of being condemned for his frailty. John Smith may have been criticized by others for failing to cope with life; but he may legitimately hope that the therapist will not readily add his own criticisms to those of others. In proclaiming this philosophy the therapist is not unique. There are many in society who also believe that the admission of weakness is not shameful, but usually they do not, like the therapist, publicly identify themselves as holders of this viewpoint. (The psychotherapeutic situation is therefore an ambiguous one in respect of shame. In becoming a 'patient' John Smith risks shame for doing so, yet seeks a place where relief from shame appears a possibility.)

5. Psychotherapy, along with some other professions, offers a possible meaning when a person has lost faith in the meanings around him. John Smith may have little faith that the therapist can help him (and his family may think likewise), but he has now – perhaps as a last resort – placed himself in a novel situation with a person who appears to have some hope that, given time, there is the possibility of making sense. (The ease with which he first turns to the therapist will depend both on the degree of his disillusionment

with the meanings of society and on the stance which he perceives the therapist to take in relation to these meanings.)

6. He may need to confide in someone who has no power over him, who is not his parent, boss, or teacher or their agent, who will not report him to other people, or side with them against him, who is free from the pressure of the family or state to mould him in a certain direction, who has no axe to grind, who is committed to confidentiality, who will make no demands upon him other than a reward for the time spent working with him and those demands which will spontaneously arise during the course of the encounter.

7. He may not have the courage to seek out anyone as a friend and confidant unless given the implicit permission to do so by a situation such as the therapeutic one. In this setting he is allowed to approach another person, a stranger, with the implication that the latter has an interest in him. He does not have to take the risk (which might be quite impossible for him) of making the usual social movements by means of which people reach out for friendship. I am not here assuming that he expects an experience as rich as friendship from the therapist, nor that the therapist will offer it or even feel it is the appropriate thing to offer, but the patient may be able to expect some degree of interest beyond the cursory, and probably carries within him, even if unconsciously, a hope of the deepest intimacy. (It is a measure of the lack of intimacy in our society that the patient so often reaches the therapist with such a desperate urge for it and with such difficulty in finding it elsewhere.)

8. The therapist, at least at the beginning, implicitly conveys that he does not expect his own emotional needs to be met in the encounter. (As the relationship develops there can be exceptions to this: occasions when the most important factor for both participants is that the 'patient' helps the 'therapist'.) Thus someone who feels empty and useless is relieved of the responsibility – which might be intolerable to him – of forcing himself to be the person he imagines the therapist wishes him to be. He is permitted a kind of freedom that he could not easily find elsewhere.

9. If a person turns to another (a friend or relative) for help, the latter may, if the problem is difficult, feel inadequate for the task. Although such misgivings may arise too readily (we all too easily seek an 'expert') yet the humility may be both understandable and justified. The psychotherapist – although his ability to help may depend upon rather different factors than those which the layman

The Situation of Psychotherapy 41

assumes to be important – not only has experience of similar situations but an implicit permission to offer his help. He has set himself up as a person who will 'take on' apparently insoluble problems, without necessarily guaranteeing success. The therapist does not have to face the nagging question 'Should I call in the "expert"?' He *is* the expert.

We cannot, however, leave the matter without an attempt to understand what is meant by the word 'expert' in this context. If the psychotherapist has to rely primarily on his ordinary human qualities and experiences in what sense can he be called an expert?

People not uncommonly drift into the role of therapist long before they would use the word to describe their function. They are those to whom friends intuitively turn for help when distressed. Although it would surely be inadvisable for one such person to put up his professional plate without first turning to those experienced in this work to guide and teach him, let us imagine that he does just this. He finds a room in which to work and his first patient arrives. Already, without any training or experience, he is in a slightly different position, in view of his commitment, from the man-in-the-street. He has made the decision to take on this role, and even before the patient arrives he has thought about the situation. And he will be in the state of mind in which he accepts the responsibility – as an 'expert' should – of his part in this particular situation, one that is not quite like any other in life. As he progresses, he will draw not only on his own increasing experience but on the experience of others – past and present – who have trodden the same path. And so he will become an expert not only because of the role he chooses to adopt but by his familiarity with it. But although his expertise is unique it has sufficient in common with other experiences of living with people (in particular, situations such as parent/child or teacher/pupil in which one person seeks to enable another to grow) to ensure that the greatest part of his capacity to help is learned in the 'school of life'; or, to put it another way, his capacity to help depends more on being able to apply a realistic experience of ordinary living to the special situation of psychotherapy than on any other factor. If he comes to believe that the efficacy of his specialized experience or that the rigours of his scientific theory and technique can supplant or transcend the application of his ordinary experience of people, then the whole endeavour is threatened.

No one can live a perfectly balanced life, with equal competence in all fields. We are, in a sense, all experts in certain matters; we have all specialized in various ways, whether we term this professional or not. The urgency which underlies my confrontation of this matter comes from the fear (based on observation) that in areas, such as psychotherapy, which involve a striving towards intimacy with, and understanding of, people, there is a pervasive and insidious tendency to avoid actual experience and replace it with a more limited and impoverished framework of thought.

I have suggested that the circumstances in which therapy takes place are very favourable and make the task of the therapist much easier than it might be for those around the patient in his normal living conditions. Moreover, if the personal factor in the encounter is crucial then it will seem less one between expert and novice than between two equals both of whom bring their experience of living to the set-up. The therapist is therefore not alone in his endeavour to reach the other; rather, two people are reaching for each other and, in such a situation, help will not necessarily be only one-way. But mutuality of this kind is something that is likely to develop over a period of time. At the beginning of therapy, or when a consultation is made at a time of crisis, the position of the therapist as professed expert can be very comforting to the patient. And, indeed, the therapist's task is sometimes made so easy by his position that he has to do little more than avoid stupidity. I will give an example of this.

Recently a woman came to see me who, two weeks previously, in the middle of a savage civil war, had left her country. On arriving in England, she had broken down and become extremely depressed. She could speak no English at all and brought her teenage daughter with her to act as interpreter.

I said very little to her. Not only was there the problem of translation, but the complicated feelings she had about her country were difficult to understand in a short space of time; I did not know enough about her relationship with her daughter to avoid possible dangerous ground between them, and, finally, the woman cried for most of the session. What I did say was of a reassuring nature. In particular I made the comment that I did not think she was seriously ill. At the end of the session the woman smiled at me and said, via her daughter, 'I feel much better'.

The fact that this patient saw me as an 'expert' (and therefore different from her relatives and friends in England) was a consolation and helped towards the integration which she subsequently managed without professional aid, but the crucial element in my reaction was, I think, that I was not too disturbed by her in spite of showing sympathy with her plight, and I did not condemn or despise her. It is likely that the confidence I have gained from experience of being with those in a state of grief conveyed itself to her in a comforting way. But I believe I was enormously helped by the sheer fact of the 'professional' setting and I would have had to behave in a very silly way to have messed up the interview.

By contrast let us consider a non-facilitating setting in which, nevertheless, people sometimes disclose their problems to someone outside their family and intimate friends. I was once consulted by a man who gave as a reason (among several others) for his anxiety the fact that his clients' problems were getting him down. He was a hairdresser. Because he was a master of his craft he had regular customers, many of whom came some distance to see him and the 'sessions' were of comparable time to those of a psychotherapist. Moreover, the content of the sessions was not entirely dissimilar for his clients made good use of his listening ear. He did his best both with their hair and their torment. 'I am', he said ruefully, 'the cheapest psychiatrist in London.' But for all his sensitivity he lacked many things, and most of all he lacked the kind of setting and assumptions which would make rigorous therapy possible. In his place, with his experience, I would cry out for a book by Freud or Jung. But, even more, I would miss my quiet room, the absence of scissors, the sense of focus and purpose, and someone to whom I could bring *my* problems.

To look at therapy in this way is to emphasize what should not be – what should be *absent* from the setting. One also has to consider what should be absent from the therapist's responses – what he should not do. The following would seem relevant. The therapist should not, in a polite or conventional way, smooth over difficulties or (worse) humour the patient or adopt a patronizing bedside manner; nor should he be committed to the opposite dogma – a relentless pursuit of the truth at all costs on all occasions, with an accompanying need to open up old wounds in the interests of theoretical rigour; his primary aim should not be to understand the patient, nor to learn from him, nor to enlarge the frontiers of science through his studies of him, nor to obtain friendship to assuage his own loneliness or to seek a substitute for child, spouse, parent, or lover. He should not use the patient to treat, vicariously, his own neurosis or as a captive audience for his own particular brand of theory. He should be able to take the risk that the patient may disturb him profoundly and he must be prepared to weather his own feelings of guilt, shame, failure, rejection, or loss without trying to turn the tables on the patient from the strength of his own position.

This list could be fruitfully extended, but already it would appear that it is easier for a camel to go through the eye of a needle than for someone to set himself up, with justification and confidence, as a therapist. But, however daunting, these requirements remain within the compass of what we might call ordinary personal endeavour. If this view of things is justified then psychotherapy is both more difficult and easier than is usually thought to be the case; it is simply that the capacities required are drawn from a much wider – perhaps infinitely wide – source than either the profession or the public at present appreciate.

The perspective that I am here proposing for psychotherapy is, therefore, embarrassingly unspecific. It becomes increasingly difficult to know what one can say about the subject, beyond the fact that it refers to a situation in which one person is aiming to help another to grow by offering him a relationship that has much in common with those in ordinary living but takes place in an unusual context. It is illusory in that, however genuine the relationship, it occurs in a setting designed to promote intimacy without distracting factors, but although it may easily be overlooked how protective this environment is, one must also remember that all relationships exclude some areas of reality and thereby foster illusion. It is as elemental and varied as, say, that between friends, lovers, marriage partners, or parents and children. It will be creative, sterile, or destructive according to the degree to which certain virtues enter into the relationship; and what is or is not a virtue is, of course, a question to which man has sought an answer since the beginning of history and for which there appears to be no foreseeable consensus of opinion, being the eternal enigma: 'How should we live?' There are no definable, formal qualifications that enable one to practise psychotherapy or even to define the aims of therapy. We can only give an opinion that certain human qualities and certain experiences are likely to be helpful.

What, then, can be usefully said? In the first place, if I have the humility to recognize that I cannot hope to produce a formula for living, and that one cannot tell another person how to practise psychotherapy, then I can perhaps within these limits say something about my experiences, and deductions from them, which might help others. And, in the second place, given the present viewpoint on the nature of psychotherapy, there is an obvious and formidable task to be confronted: to show the manner in which established theoretical formulations about psychotherapy either enhance or hinder creative practice, and to find a way of encompassing the fact that practitioners working within frameworks which depart significantly from that which would appear desirable have handed down invaluable truths to us – the most obvious example, and by far the most challenging, being that of Freud and those who have derived their inspiration from his work. In other words, we have to ask ourselves whether the practice of psychotherapy requires us to rely on a specialized theory developed in the last century involving new ideas about human nature, its development, its pathology and the healing of its pathology, or whether there is an alternative way of formulating what we do (and whether or not to call this alternative a theory).

Within the framework that I have outlined a therapist will, in the course of time, learn a great deal about how he himself and those who come to him experience and act in that framework. If he were gifted enough he would, I believe, discover a significant amount of the richness that is to be found, from Freud onwards, in the writings of those who have worked in this way. But the greater part of his learning will take the form of improvement in his intuitive response. As Rycroft[1] has pointed out, although Freud saw himself as an objective scientist who worked by the use of theory, in practice he neither engaged the patient in this way nor advocated that one should do so: rather he suggested that the analyst be open to the patient with 'free-floating attention'. This means that he relied primarily on his intuition – an attribute acquired in his ordinary living which he then brought to a novel setting. The point at which one can justifiably speak of perceiving according to theory is an arbitrary one, for we are bound to structure our world by means of expectations which, even in primitive form, could perhaps be called theories. Knowledge in a specialized area of experience (the psychotherapeutic set-up) can improve the accuracy of our expectations but, should the latter derive mainly from this knowledge, then we would be working according to theory in the usual sense of that phrase. It is by no means certain that psychotherapists do work in this way; it is even less certain that they should, and if they do then their procedure is best described by the particular theory in question (e.g. psychoanalysis, bio-energetics, etc.). Those of us who subscribe to a non-technical way of practising psychotherapy may hope to make observations (which could be called piecemeal theories) but not to build a theory of the enterprise.

Is this eclectism? Not, I believe, in the sense in which the term is normally used. Eclecticism implies that one investigates the various schools of thought and builds up a theory which incorporates differing viewpoints into a balanced whole. But in fact it would take a genius to do this. How, for instance, could one solve the incompatibilities between Kleinian and Behaviourist theories without years of philosophical deliberation? Eclecticism, to my mind, is a myth. Psychotherapists have the choice between espousing one particular theory or basing their work on an over-all philosophical view of living (which includes their attitude to healing) and then modifying their chosen framework under the influence of new experience, either direct or learned from the insights of others (some of which will be expressed in an alien framework of thought). What I aim to explore in this book is the idea that not only is it possible to conceive of a psychotherapy based on a view of living derived primarily from ordinary experience but that such a psychotherapy offers the most realistic and useful framework available to us.

We are living at a certain period of history and cannot forget this. It affects our conception of psychotherapy in two ways. Firstly, the kinds of problems which patients bring to us will depend to some extent on the kind of problems to which our society, at this time, is subject, and we cannot avoid taking the latter into consideration. Secondly, the practice of any discipline is affected by the creative innovations of genius and by fashion, bringing changes which, whether constructive or not, will necessarily have to be confronted before they can be assimilated or discarded. In the field of psychotherapy the innovation of the greatest import has been an emphasis upon the personal history of those who are troubled and we are now faced with the task of incorporating the insights derived from this approach into the general philosophy of our practice.

Although psychotherapy and art are profoundly different in some ways, the two pursuits share certain important features. They are both concerned with the pursuit of truth in the personal realm and the search for ways by means of which it can be communicated. There is reason to believe that the field of art contains a challenge comparable to the one I have just suggested in psychotherapy.

The American poet, Richard Wilbur, writing about his own work, suggests that, early in this century, a new creative force entered American poetry, through the work of Frost, Robinson, Sandburg, Pound, Eliot, Stein, Cummings, and others:

Another question often asked of the poets of my generation is where do they stand in relation to the revolution in American poetry which is said to have begun in the second decade of this century. I think that there truly was a revolution then in poetry as in the other arts, and if one looks at poetry anthologies of the year 1900 one can see that a revolution was called for – a revolution against trivial formalism, dead rhetoric, and genteel subject matter. The revolution was not a concerted one and there was little agreement on objectives; nor is there now any universal agreement as to what, in that revolution, was most constructive. But certainly it has been of lasting importance that Robinson and Frost chose to enliven traditional metres with the rhythms of colloquial speech; that Sandburg and others insisted on slang and on the brute facts of the urban and industrial scene; and that Pound and Eliot sophisticated American verse by introducing techniques from other literatures, and by reviving and revising our sense of literary tradition.

But Wilbur is determined that, however much he has gained from these innovations, however much he cannot avoid their idiom, he will not allow them to detract from the total experience of living and working:

We have seen, in this century, a number of the arts entrapped in reductive theories: music, some have said, is merely sound in time; architecture is nothing but the provision of areas for living or working; painting is only the arrangement of line and colour on a plain surface. All these definitions are true enough, except for those words 'merely' and 'only' and 'nothing but', which imply that to go beyond the bare fundamentals of any art is to risk impurity. There have been, as I have said, a number of reductive approaches to poetry in this century, but somehow American poetry has never fallen into such a condition as we now find American painting, where for the most part one must choose between the solipsism of abstract expressionism and the empty objectivity of so-called pop art.

My own position on poetry, if I have to have one, is that it should include every resource which can be made to work. Aristotle, as you may remember, argued that drama is the highest of the arts because it contains more means and elements than any other. I am not sure that Aristotle is right about the pre-eminence of drama, but I do share his feeling that an art should contain as much as it can and still be itself. As a poet, my relationship to the revolution in question is that I am the grateful inheritor of all that my talent can employ, but that I will not accept any limitations or prohibitions or exclude anything in the name of purity. So far as possible, I try to play the whole instrument.[2]

As psychotherapists we are, I think, in a similar position in regard to the movement, derived from Freud and those who have followed his thought closely, which draws our attention to the importance of personal history. Not only would we be stupid to try to ignore it; we cannot do so. But we must now, after the overwhelming impact of its force, try to regain our balance. And we must do this less by emphasizing the opposite to the historical approach – the 'here-and-now' situation in the encounter – than by giving more weight to the ordinary unspecialized features of helping than is at present customary, *i.e. to searching out features which are intrinsic to the helping situation – without imposing formulations derived from theories that centre upon one particular element in experience (e.g. birth, conditioned reflex, confrontation, sexuality, muscular tension, interpretation, objectivity, dependence, shock tactics, and so on).* Let us therefore now take a look at the personal historical approach and try to establish the degree to which it should inform our work.

References

1. Rycroft, C. (1977), The Present State of Psychoanalysis, broadcast talk on BBC Radio 3, 21 October 1977.
2. Wilbur, R. (1976), *Responses*, Harcourt Brace Jovanovich, New York.

4. The Paradox of Transference

'Why are you sighing?'
'For all the voyages I did not make
Because the boat was small, might leak, might take
The wrong course, and the compass might be broken,
And I might have awakened
In some strange sea and heard
Strange birds crying.'

'Why are you weeping?'
'For all the unknown friends and lovers passed
Because I watched the ground or walked too fast
Or simply did not see
Or turned aside for tea
For fear an old wound stirred
From its sleeping.' – A. S. J. Tessimond, 'Talk in the Night'

This morning a woman in her thirties told me that yesterday she had received a letter from her mother who lived several hundred miles away and whom she saw only now and again. The very sight of the letter disturbed her and it was several hours before she could bring herself to open it. I report this incident not because it is unusual but because it is the kind of occurrence that is so common. It is a measure of the impact of the past. This woman circled round the letter as though it were a bomb. And, in a sense, it was, for it contained the accumulated power of thirty years' experience, the greatest intensity of which was furthest from the present. It is this power which Freud has brought to our notice with such force and precision. No discussion of therapy can afford to omit the concept which he referred to as 'transference'.

In this book I have aimed to dispense with special terminology and have sought to show that we need not look beyond the ordinary to find the basis of our practice, but it seems perverse to try to bypass the word used by Freud himself for the idea which has brought us so much understanding. The phenomenon of transference appears to me to be the one feature of psychotherapeutic practice that is so little knowingly experienced in ordinary living, so little taken into account (despite the fact that it occurs) in ordinary living, that we are justified in saying that, in this case, twentieth-century psychotherapy has added a new dimension to the possibilities of helping people. This does not mean that a knowledge of transference is a substitute for all the unspecialized ways in which people may help each other but it does imply that those who study and practise in this field of endeavour would be extraordinarily misled if they failed to take full cognizance of its existence.

Our conception of the present is largely a product of our past. We have a realistic expectation that the kind of experiences which have previously occurred are likely to be repeated. Without this expectation we would be utterly lost. To this extent we *transfer* earlier experiences on to our present perceptual field.

The term transference, as used by psychoanalysts, has come to refer to inappropriate expectations derived from past experiences. There are several reasons why a person may gain a wrong impression of a situation. He may, for instance, have been given some false information. It is when the reason for the distortion lies in a persuasive tendency to misperceive because he remains so much under the influence of past events – particularly those of childhood – that we are justified in using the term transference in the sense given to it by psychoanalysts.

Greenson and Wexler define the term thus:

Transference is the experiencing of impulses, feelings, fantasies, attitudes, and defences with respect to a person in the present which do not appropriately fit that person but are a repetition of responses originating in regard to significant persons of early childhood, unconsciously displaced on to persons in the present. The two outstanding characteristics of transference phenomena are (1) it is an indiscriminate, non-selective repetition of the past, and (2) it ignores or distorts reality. It is inappropriate.[1]

The usefulness of carefully noting the ways in which the patient distorts his perception of the therapist cannot be denied, and the emotional intensity and incredible persistence of some of these distortions would, I believe, come as a great surprise to those not accustomed to experiencing them (either as therapist or patient) in the therapeutic setting. Let us take a closer look at the concept.

The basic learning in the past concerns the nature of persons (including the self) and the best way in which to relate to them. It derives from direct experience but is conditional on two distinct facets: the universal (what the human animal is like) and the social (what people in one's own society are like). Let us assume that the patient approaches the therapist with expectations derived from both his experience of people and his knowledge and assumptions about the professional role of the therapist, and let us, for the moment, set aside the latter (the anticipation of the 'technical' moves of the therapist). One realistic expectation on the patient's part would be that the therapist is unique, that it would take a while to understand him, and that his first judgements may have to be reviewed: in other words, the patient's perception would be flexible and would allow for growth in the relationship. An inappropriate expectation would reveal itself in a judgement that is too quick.

The essence, therefore, of the kind of transference manifestations that interest the therapist is *rigidity*. Moreover, it is always, I believe, accompanied by an expectation of a reciprocal rigidity on the part of the therapist. How can the latter help his patient to overcome the problem? It is useful – and current practice – to point out these rigidities to the patient. But it would seem reasonable to suggest that the *sine qua non* of any approach is flexibility. Let me give an example.

A young woman has recently started coming to see me. One day she arrived a little late, was reluctant to talk, and seemed, in a not obvious way, somewhat cross with me. After a while she told me she had felt hurt after the previous session because I appeared to be critical of her intimate revelations. One particular comment of mine had upset her: I had said, 'You seem to be treating me like a father confessor.'

In fact I had not felt critical of the content of her revelations but of the manner in which she made them. She appeared to be presenting a list of all the bad things she had done and dutifully presenting them to me as though I required her to do so, and I thought that she was transferring on to me an image from her past.

After we had talked of this further I said: 'You *are* making me feel something: I feel that I have to treat you very carefully, very gently, or you will get hurt.'

She appeared at first to accept this but still looked negative and troubled. Then I said: 'It's difficult, isn't it? I'm not sure whether you are a very vulnerable person, whether you cast yourself in that role for defensive purposes, or whether I was a bit clumsy and you want to have that accepted.'

'I think it's the last,' she said. 'I was just pouring out things I'd never said to anyone. I just wanted you to listen. I didn't want you to say what you did. I'm sorry. I don't expect you to be perfect, and I don't expect you not to criticize me. It's just that it was wrong for me at that moment.'

During this discussion I had made what is usually called a transference interpretation: that is to say, I had assumed in her, from the
basis of my own response and my perception of my own behaviour
to her, that she was projecting on to me an undue expectation of
hurtful actions. But I think I was wrong. This short interchange is an
example of the ease with which the conception of transference can
so easily lead one to make unjustified criticisms. It may be thought –
especially by those for whom the notion of transference dominates
their work – that I was right first time and wrong now: that the
patient manoeuvred me into defeat. I do not think that this was so,
but what I believe is that something more important happened.
From that moment an atmosphere began to develop in which the
question of who was right or wrong in any particular matter did not
dominate our transactions – we came to trust each other's flexibility. This recognition showed itself in her sigh of relief, the gratitude
of her smile, and the subsequent and lasting improvement in our
relationship. An ideal of flexibility can of course be an excuse for
vacillation and weakness: as in most matters one can be wrong in
opposite kinds of ways. But the justification for an emphasis on
flexibility lies not only in the above argument but in the fact that,
when the therapist disagrees with the patient, the former's reliance
on the concept of transference to validate his own viewpoint is a less
impressive court of appeal than he usually assumes it to be.

It is when we are faced with a difference in ways of being or
philosophical outlook that the concept is at its most vulnerable
point, for the patient has to make an adequate assessment of the
therapist's limitations. If, for instance, a patient is reticent or, by
contrast, demonstrative, are these inappropriate reactions to the
therapeutic situation (i.e. manifestations of transference) or are
they ways of being that are individual but reasonable and acceptable? We are here in the midst of the question concerning the
distinction between health and sickness. And, to the degree that
this problem defies a satisfactory solution, it is clear that transference interpretations have their limits and must be used with
caution. The patient is dependent on the therapist's realistic grasp
of living and it may be no better than his own. If we are to protect
the patient from this kind of error (idealization of the therapist's
perception of reality), transference must be given second place to a
mutual exploration of each other's stance.

No one has recognized this danger more clearly than Szasz, and his instructive essay 'The Concept of Transference' has not received the attention it deserves. He writes:

The concept of transference serves two separate analytic purposes: it is a crucial part of the patient's therapeutic experience, and a successful defensive measure to protect the analyst from too intense affective and real-life involvement with the patient. For the idea of transference implies denial and repudiation of the patient's *experience qua experience*; in its place is substituted the more manageable construct of a *transference experience*.

Thus if the patient loves or hates the analyst, and if the analyst can view these attitudes as transference, then, in effect, the analyst has convinced himself that the patient does not have these feelings and disposition towards *him*. The patient does not really love or hate the analyst, but someone else. This is why so-called transference interpretations are so easily and so often misused; they provide a ready-made opportunity for putting the patient at arm's length.[2]

Szasz is here concerned with a special kind of transference, namely a 'too intensive affective one' (which psychoanalysts call 'positive' or 'negative'). This form of transference is often referred to in a colloquial manner, by professional and layman alike, as synonymous with the concept itself. Thus the person who comes to his therapist and says 'I suppose I am expected to get a transference on you', really means 'I suppose I am expected to fall in love with you'. The reasons for this kind of assumption are primarily historical ones and follow from Freud's early experience with women patients. Szasz's observations on one item of history – the relationship between Freud, Breuer, Anna O., and Freud's wife – are illuminating on this point.

Breuer fled in alarm from the advances of the patient Anna O. and relinquished his interest in the matter, whereas Freud, who had no personal therapeutic relationship with her, continued to explore the meaning of it all and conceived the notion of 'transference', thereby removing the threat of being the object of an attractive woman's yearning. Szasz notes, however, that before protecting himself by this intellectual conviction he first felt the need to reassure his wife that, for such a thing to happen, 'one has to be a Breuer'. Szasz ends his paper thus:

The concept of transference was reassuring for another reason as well. It introduced into medicine and psychology the notion of the *therapist as a symbol*: this renders the *therapist as person* essentially invulnerable.

When an object becomes a symbol (of another object) people no longer react to it as an object; hence, its features *qua* object become inscrutable. Consider the flag as the symbol of the nation. It may be defiled, captured by the enemy, even destroyed; national identity which the flag symbolizes, lives on nevertheless.

The concept of transference performs a similar function, the analyst is only a symbol (therapist), for the object he represents (internal image). If, however, the therapist is accepted as symbol – say of the father – his specific individuality becomes inconsequential. As the flag, despite what happens to it, remains a symbol of the nation, so the analyst, regardless of what he does, remains a symbol of the father to the patient. Herein lies the danger. Just as the pre-Freudian physician was ineffective partly because he remained a fully 'real' person, so the psycho-analyst may be ineffective if he remains a fully 'symbolic' object. The analytic situation requires the therapist to function as both, and the patient to perceive him as both. Without these conditions, 'analysis' cannot take place.

The use of the concept of transference in psychotherapy thus led to two different results. On the one hand, it enabled the analyst to work where he could not otherwise have worked; on the other, it exposed him to the danger of being 'wrong' vis-a-vis his patient – and of abusing the analytic relationship without anyone being able to demonstrate this to him.[3]

There is, in fact, an increasing recognition by psychoanalysts that a 'real' relationship exists in addition to the transference. This has led to the idea known as the 'working alliance':

The 'working alliance' is the non-neurotic, rational, reasonable rapport which the patient has with his analyst and which enables him to work purposefully in the analytic situation despite his transference impulses.[4]

However, this concept is a makeshift operation which ensures that the 'non-transference' remains a necessary but uninteresting and *uninvestigated* phenomenon within the context of which the important things happen. Thereby wholeness is lost; the relationship is artificially divided into two distinct parts for the sake of theoretical convenience and – probably – tranquillity of mind. We need therefore to explore the matter further.

When two people meet in a setting liable to promote intimacy there are two different modes, other than that of simple friendship, in which they may unconsciously visualize the relationship: as parent/child or as lovers. Although the patient may wish to act as parent to the therapist this is an aim that is far removed from the overt agreement and, if present, is likely to emerge only gradually and indirectly. Therefore we are left with two likely configurations:

1. The patient is looking for a parent.
2. The patient is looking for a lover.

It is a paradox that the method of treatment that is noted – and even castigated – for its emphasis on sexuality should in one particular way evade it. I refer to the fact that the psychoanalyst does not readily assume that his patient seeks a lover. If, indeed, there are signs that such may be the case, he is likely to say: 'You seek in me the parent with whom you wanted a sensuous or sexual relationship.' In other words, he fails to recognize that the therapeutic set-up is one which may easily engender a wish to be treated as a lover. In such a situation the therapist is not a symbol for the patient: he is a sexual being. For this reason it is not so easy to dismiss the patient's feelings as projections or transference phenomena. But can they still be regarded as artefacts?

Love for another person does not exist outside a context. There are always elements, real or illusory, temporary or permanent, which are likely to evoke or inhibit the emergence of love. There is (it seems to me) something especially 'real' in a love which lasts, which survives the rigours of time and trouble. But it would be a hard (and I believe mistaken) man who would dismiss as illusory all love feelings which derive their force from certain moments in time, certain stages in life, or certain happy circumstances. What is impermanent is not necessarily inauthentic.

Despite the fact that the therapeutic situation is transient (although it may last for years) and derives some of its meaning from unusually facilitating circumstances, we should not dismiss the feelings aroused as necessarily bogus, nor attempt to support this criticism by resort to the theory of transference. But we should surely take full cognizance of all those factors – including transference – leading to a surge of emotions which, whether authentic or not, may distort our view of the truth and seriously disturb our lives.

Protection from such temptation comes, of course, not only from ourselves but our patients. The degree of intimacy that each partner desires, feels appropriate, and is willing to risk is, I believe, worked out carefully (if largely unconsciously) by both people from the beginning of the relationship. And it is done not simply by the 'technique' of the therapist and the 'inhibitions' of the patient but by those delicate and primarily non-verbal signs by which people declare their degree of interest in, trust of, and sense of responsibility towards each other. Judgements of this kind tend to escape accounts of psychotherapeutic work. It is difficult for me to find examples either in my own experience or that of others. But a brief description of the sort of dilemma to which a psychotherapist is frequently exposed may be useful.

Ruth sought my help because of sudden 'black-outs' for which no organic cause could be found. In spite of her alarming symptoms she approached me without any apparent sense of urgency. We arranged for her to have sessions three times a week. After four weeks I had to be away for a few days and we consequently missed two sessions. I had given her due warning of this. Up to the point of the break we had been getting on rather well; she was keen to come and alert when with me. But on my return she spoke of her reluctance to be here, the irritation of the long journey, the thought that she might crash her car. Then she told me that on waking up this morning she was aware of a dream or fantasy in which she was nailing me down in a coffin. During our discussions of these thoughts she realized that, to her surprise, she felt deeply hurt by my brief absence, to a degree that accounted for the dream. This sequence of events indicates the rapidity and intensity with which strong feelings can be aroused – even by a therapist who has not deliberately designed a setting for the purpose of their arousal. And, because the intensity is so inappropriate it is hard to avoid the conclusion that the simple fact of coming for help has stirred up some of the feelings of dependence, loss, and fury that occurred in her childhood.

Two weeks later Ruth told me about a dream in which she came for her session but was dismayed to find that another man was present. In her dream I said to her: 'This man, who is a psychotherapist, is seeing you today instead of me'. She was enraged: 'But I don't want just a psychotherapist, I want Peter Lomas'. Her only thought about the other man was that 'there was something official about him'.

At first sight this could again be interpreted as a transference dream. Ruth was being reminded of the times in childhood when her loved parent was replaced by a stranger and she was expected to accept the replacement. No doubt such occurrences were painful and left their mark. But, before making interpretations based on well-established lines of thought, one might ask whether the main reference of the dream is to the present rather than to the past. Ruth came to me with the assumption that our relationship would be a formal one and up to that point I had made little of an attempt to steer her into more informal waters. My own reading of the dream is that she is expressing her wish for a less professional, more personal encounter. And, although this in turn could have transference implications (referring to memories of a lack of intimacy between herself and her parents) I am inclined to the view that Ruth's dream asks the question, 'What kind of intimacy is desirable and possible in this situation?'

A week or so later Ruth reported another dream. She was walking with a certain actor and they were becoming increasingly attracted to each other. They began to fondle each other and then the man's wife appeared on the scene. However, far from criticizing them, the wife appeared embarrassed and withdrew, having apologized for interrupting procedures. Later in the dream, together with the man, she was searching for a bowl, said to be beautiful, which must be rescued from the hands of wicked people aiming to possess it. She succeeded in finding the bowl and hid it in a lake where it would be safe. There was a feeling of pleasure in sharing this act. The bowl was made of pewter and was not beautiful, but she had the thought, 'It must have value even if I cannot see this myself'. At one point in the dream she said to herself, 'It is strange. I feel close to this man but we have not gone to bed together'.

Ruth thought that the man represented me and the bowl represented herself. Of the actor she said that he had recently appeared in two plays both of which involved triangular situations. In one of these a married woman had an affair in which it was not clear whether the two people slept together or discussed in detail the fantasy of sleeping together.

Ruth did not describe the second play in which the actor had appeared but I happened to have seen it myself and I remembered that there was one scene between a man and a much younger woman which had provoked incestuous fantasies in me. I mentioned this to Ruth who responded by reminding me that her own father had behaved in a provocatively sexual way towards her when she was a child.

It seems fairly clear that the dream is about Ruth's loving and sexual feelings towards me, of which she is unconscious, and her wishes that I respond. The latter part of the dream refers, I think, to her hope that she and I will find her true self and share it in a way that will convince her that she is valuable, and her fear that sharing of this intensity would prove disastrous. But the questions relevant to this discussion are: 'Why does she feel such loving, sexual feelings for me? Why does she need to repress them? What am I to say to her about her revelations?'

In fact I interpreted these feelings as a transference of her incestuous urges towards her father. But, on reflection, I am not sure that I was right in laying such emphasis on the past. I think that Ruth dealt with her embarrassment at the possibility of mutual attraction by repressing her feelings for me and when they were revealed I colluded with her and spared my own embarrassment by gratefully resorting to the psychoanalytic theory that such emotions are artefacts, dramatizations of events that occurred safely in the past and hold no dangers in the present: in short, that they were *merely* transference phenomena.

Acting on this thought I discussed with Ruth the temptations and anxieties to which we were both subject because of our intimate situation. I did not until later admit in words that I found her attractive. Following this interchange the dreams ceased; the crisis was over and the therapy proceeded to a satisfactory conclusion a few months later.

I do not, however, take it for granted that this discussion was crucial. Rather I suspect that a silent agreement was made between us by means of our non-verbal behaviour. The consulting room in which I worked at that time was relatively small. In order to get to the door, Ruth had to pass quite close to me; as she did so we usually looked at each other and smiled. I often felt an impulse to touch her at this moment, but never did so. I think that our smiles conveyed a message which, if put into words, would be, 'I like you but such attraction that I feel is within manageable bounds. I want to keep it that way and I believe you do also. Therefore we know where we stand.'

Is this silent agreement merely a 'working alliance'? I think not. The tentative advances and consolidations in a relationship are themselves an attempt at growth. To the extent that Ruth and I are both engaged in the same process the therapy is mutual; it is an exploration of the world and of ourselves, and a sharing, which, if done with honesty, is enriching to us. (Because we are primarily concerned with Ruth's growth and not my own it is justifiable to say that *Ruth* is receiving therapy from *me*.)

The suggestion that mutual exploration and flexibility of response – comparable to the forms of fruitful relationship in ordinary life – are the key to successful therapy must not lead us to leave unexplored the reasons why therapists, by and large, have come to a rather different view. The alternative dictum is perhaps best expressed by what is known as 'The Rule of Abstinence'. In his authoritative and lucid book *The Technique and Practice of Psychoanalysis* Ralph Greenson spells out the conditions for 'safeguarding the transference' so the patient 'can develop the greatest variety and intensity of transference reactions in accordance with his own, unique individual history and his own needs'. In a section entitled 'The Rule of Abstinence', he writes:

Freud made the important recommendation that the treatment should be carried out, as far as possible, with the patient in a state of abstinence. He stated very clearly: 'Analytic treatment should be carried through, as far as is possible, under privation – in a state of abstinence'. 'Cruel though it may sound,' he added 'we must see to it that the patient's suffering, to a degree that is in some way or other effective, does not come to an end prematurely! The patient's symptoms, which drove him into treatment, consist in part of warded-off instincts seeking satisfaction. These instinctual impulses will turn to the analyst and the analytic situation as long as the analyst consistently avoids offering the patient substitute gratifications. The prolonged frustration will induce the patient to regress, so that his entire neurosis will be re-experienced in the transference, the transference neurosis. However, allowing symptom-substitute gratifications of any magnitude, in or outside of the analytic situation, will rob the patient of his neurotic suffering and his motivations to continue treatment'.

The rule of abstinence has been misunderstood and misconstrued to mean that the patient was prohibited from enjoying any instinctual gratification during the analysis. Actually Freud was trying to prevent the patient from making a premature 'flight into health' and effecting a so called 'transference cure'.

In order to ensure the maintenance of adequate motivation, (a) it is necessary for the psychoanalyst consistently to point out to the patient the infantile and unrealistic quality of the instinctual satisfaction which the patient is attempting to obtain, and (b) to make sure that the analyst is in no way consciously or unconsciously gratifying the patient's infantile neurotic instinctual needs.[5]

Greenson is well known for his flexibility. Other writers can be more stringent. In the *International Review of Psychoanalysis*, Serge Viderman makes a clear and uncompromising statement of Freudian technique:

To the patient's smiles, to his small talk, the analyst has firmly and tenaciously offered a particular, specific reception. He has maintained the necessary distance unchanged, he has deliberately kept the stereotyped solemnity of the encounter. He has answered most remarks of the patient with silence, parsimonious replies, or the calculated tone of interpretation . . .

Perhaps it is now time to draw up the list of rules which govern the analytic field:

(1) The fixed and non-interchangeable positions of the *physical* space of the analysis;
(2) The two fundamental rules –
        for the couch: free association;
        for the armchair: evenly sustained attention.
(3) Neutrality;
(4) Benevolence;
(5) The specificity of the encounter;
(6) The required speech of one;
(7) The professional silence of the other;
(8) The passivity of the analyst, altered only by his interpretations.

This set of interdependent rules constitutes the specific foundation of what we believe to be the only conditions permitting the construction of an analytic space and the unfolding of an authentic psychoanalytic process; without them we may be in the presence of various other psychotherapeutic acts – but not of genuine psychoanalysis.

Later, Viderman compares the patient in analysis with the people enclosed in Plato's cave:

Their situation in the space of the cave, with necks in the pillory, unable to turn round, is not without a striking analogy to our situation in the analytic space. For we too (because the very rules which we have set for the patient and for ourselves prohibit us from turning round), have no possibility of seeing anything except what the rules allow us to see. We have no more possibility of modifying our situation, or the rules which rigorously organise and close the space of the analysis, than do the prisoners of Plato.[6]

The imagery is striking and helps us to recognize, if we have not already done so, the crippling limitations imposed on the patient by his rigorously scientific helper. And, if I have understood Viderman correctly, he does not intend irony.

The rule of abstinence derives its justification from the belief that the crucial element in therapy is the repetition of a childhood traumatic experience in a situation which encourages a new and better resolution. To this end the therapist must create a condition which approximates to the original. There is clearly some sense in this argument; but it has been taken much too far. If someone is to overcome an anxiety or inhibition we must not make conditions so favourable that the source of his anxiety never makes its appearance on the horizon; in other words, we must not over-protect, soothe, placate, or humour him. However, if we are honest with him, and do not fall over backwards to nourish his sensitivities, then, I believe, there is little chance that he will not be faced with sufficient frustration to permit an understanding of his difficulties – certainly the possible disadvantages are small when compared to the harmful consequences of a regime *designed* to frustrate. Moreover, a non-frustrating, facilitating regime – provided it is not overprotective – would seem to be ideally suited not only to the trusting exposure of wounds but to the arousal of hope and the motivation needed for healing.

In view of the disadvantages of the rule of abstinence it is difficult to avoid the suspicion that it derives from unacknowledged forces. The first of these (which has already emerged in the discussion) is the protection of the therapist. The second is the stoical (if not puritanical) element in Freud's philosophy of living: if the medicine is to be efficacious, it must have a nasty taste.

The fact that the rule of abstinence is often applied with a crip-pling rigidity and is justified by a questionable theory does not mean, however, that some of the conventions that are practised under its name are without value. In all societies safeguards exist to prevent unwelcome, unexpected, or traumatic intrusions of priv-acy: protocol, custom, and etiquette require that certain formalities are respected before people become intimate. In Victorian times, for instance, it was considered, in high society, to be improper to approach someone without an introduction by a third party. And, although such conventions can be carried to an extreme which results in snobbery and sterility, they provide guidelines to facilitate and control the speed of development and depth of penetration of personal encounters. The 'rules' of psychoanalysis derive, I believe, primarily from the same social requirements: they are designed (unconsciously) to protect the private lives of both parties. The model on which these rules are based is that of the professional and the client, especially doctor and patient. The psychoanalyst's wife or secretary, for instance, may act as a buffer in a way that is comparable to their counterparts in a medical practice. The matter of sexuality is, however, handled differently. In place of the nurse/chaperone and the punitive legislature of the General Medical Council, the psychoanalyst has his rules of technique.

A measure designed to protect both parties should not, however, be presented in such a way as to mislead and to result in an exaggeration of the inequality of need. It is one thing for the analyst to say (putting it bluntly), 'I value my privacy and fear intrusion. Perhaps when I get to know you better I will feel safer with you and be able to show you more of myself. I see many people in a setting of intimacy and can only afford a certain amount of exposure to the penetrating gaze of others. If I am to listen to you, to focus on the problem of your life, you must not rush me, you must allow me the space I need to reflect and remain *relatively* composed. At the end of the session please go for I require a little time on my own before I meet another client . . .' and so on. But it is another thing and, to my mind, a potentially confusing one, to say, 'The fact that I keep my distance from you is nothing to do with my own personal needs and wishes. I do so because, if I were to show myself, and if I were to respond to your emotional needs instead of frustrating them, we would lose sight of your projections and fail to analyse your omnipotent infantile urges . . .'

In a therapeutic encounter a compromise will be reached in which each person decides how far he is prepared to go in revealing his own wishes and meeting the wishes of the other. The result will depend not only on the fact that this is a therapeutic set-up but on the particular needs, defences, and a sense of responsibility of the two people concerned and the degree to which they can enjoy each other's company. The repressed or ill-managed infantile urges of the client are a factor of great importance but it is mistaken to use the fact of their existence as a basis for the *design* of a therapeutic relationship. If, with certain clients, at certain moments, I restrain an impulse to touch, or to act or speak in an impulsive way, I do so less to preserve the transference than from an awareness that the intimacy of the situation requires me to move with caution – an awareness which the client may or may not share with me.

The matter of intimacy is much more subtle than the formal arrangements of therapy. We may think that touching is a sign of intimacy, yet two people can be very close to each other without touching, and distant when in each other's arms. If we are close to someone we may discern a fault, and, confident in the knowledge of our closeness, we may feel safe enough to make a criticism. Yet, on the other hand, our closeness may make us so sensitive to his state of mind that we leave our criticism to a time when he may be more responsive to it, or even keep silent in the hope that the criticism may never need to be made. The complexity of such judgements cannot easily be formulated into a theory. We can only hope that the two people concerned will find their way to a degree and kind of intimacy that enables growth to occur and is not too disturbing to either of them.

Another concept that Freud used in connection with the phenomena of repeated patterns of behaviour was 'regression'. It is a term which has given rise to much debate and some confusion and it may therefore be appropriate to consider its relation to transference.

Because all our thoughts and actions contain elements from the past and because any helping situation has its prototype in childhood, there is a sense in which it is correct to say that regression occurs during therapy. However, the concept is usually taken to denote certain experiences of a fairly well-defined nature. Regression, as understood by Freud (who was influenced by the ideas of the British physiologist, Hughlings Jackson), constitutes a defensive retreat to an infantile mode of functioning in the face of an unwelcome challenge. But in more recent years, largely under the impact, in Britain, of Winnicott and Balint, psychotherapists have come to value the state of 'therapeutic regression', a strategic and often courageous retreat, necessary in the long term if growth is to occur.[7]

The difference between transference and regression would seem to be the following. In transference a person expects matters to turn out as they have done in the past. In regression he takes an attitude to the past and to the present with special relevance to hope; he either, through hopelessness, exploits his past experience in an effort to legitimize a retreat from action, or because he hopes that a step forward is now possible (I have in mind a therapeutic setting) which will entail a return to a time when he was less neurotically equipped with protective armour and more dependent on those around him.

One final paradox. In its beginnings psychoanalysis turned away from the tenor of everyday discourse and explored the mysteries of the unconscious by means of the interpretation of dreams, free-associations, and an exploration of childhood fantasy. Later the concept of transference shifted the focus of exploration and explanation on to the here-and-now interchange in the consulting room. Thus, by a very devious route, it brought us back to the ordinary – provided, of course, we do not allow the ordinary to be lost in the obscurities of technique and theory. Let me exemplify this thought in relation to the patient I described earlier in this chapter.

Ruth came to me because of a certain symptom – 'black-outs'. But although we discussed this symptom, and its origin, from time to time, our main concern quite quickly became our relationship in the present. Could she trust me? Would I try to dominate her? Will I care about her, etc.? Thus we came to feel that the crucial issue was not her symptoms but the whole of her, and that what was most important between us was not a discussion of a symptom but an attempt to work out a relationship. I would say that what we were concerned with was not only – and not primarily – finding out whether and why she might be unduly cautious in her approach to me, nor the establishment of a trust (a 'working alliance') on the basis of which therapy can occur but the formation (or not) of a trusting relationship which in itself could be therapeutic. There were also other facets of her predicament in life which were voiced in non-medical, non-psychiatric terms. For instance, she said, 'I feel a worthless person, a burden. I have always felt like this. Sometimes I think it would have been better for others if I were dead.' Thus we were soon locked in a personal interaction, in which intuition played an enormous part. If I were to spell out in detail this approach, it would go something as follows:

'The problem which you bring me is yourself. Everything that you are manifests what is wrong with you. In your presence I shall, in time, become aware of your problem: I shall feel it because of the way that you are with me and to me. Whatever has happened to distort and cripple you is now woven into the texture of your being. You cannot conceal it if I stay with you long enough; it will emerge and I shall have a chance to understand and respond to it in a way that may be healing. Therefore, although I take note of your own formulation of the problem and will not neglect this, my main purpose will be, through my relationship with you, to get to know you better.' Such an approach is not, after all, far removed from common sense. It is a patient, circumspect line of action, which takes into consideration certain facts: in particular, that a person is not always what he says he is and that, to get to know another intimately, one must 'live' with him and see of what stuff he is made. The paradox is that, in spending my time getting to know him, I, the supposed 'specialist', find myself adopting a less specialized approach than that of a helper (whether professional or not) who focuses on his symptom and its cause and relief.

References

1. Greenson, R. and Wexler, M. (1969), 'The Nontransference Relationship in the Psychoanalytic Situation', *Int. J. Psycho-anal.* 50. 27.
2. Szasz, T. (1963), 'The Concept of Transference', *Int. J. Psycho-anal.* 44.
3. Ibid.
4. Greenson and Wexler, 'The Nontransference Relationship'.
5. Greenson, R. (1963), *The Technique and Practice of Psychoanalysis*, Hogarth, London, vol. i, p. 275.
6. Viderman, S. (1974), 'Interpretation in the Analytic Space', *Int. Rev. Psycho-anal.* 1.467.
7. Lomas, P. (1963), *True and False Experience*, Allen Lane, London.

5. Receptivity

If a dread of not being understood be hidden in the breasts
of other young people to anything like the extent to which it
used to be hidden in mine – which I consider probable, as I
have no particular reason to suspect myself of having been a
monstrosity – it is the key to many reservations. – Charles
Dickens, *Great Expectations*

To say someone is human is to make a statement about his morality:
he is less than God and therefore capable of evil, but more than a
stone and therefore capable of good. It is the good qualities which
enable him to help another, although the goodness is limited.
Whereas religion helps through the intervention of God,
psychotherapy relies on the frailty of a human being. But this frailty
is not all loss, for the sufferer may feel less awed by – and therefore
less defensive towards – someone who shows himself in his true
colours, even if the colours are a bit faded.

In this chapter I will try to give a picture of the way I was with
someone who come to me for help. The account will inevitably be
arbitrary for, to the extent that I reveal myself rather than pursue a
method, the encounter will have as much in common with, say, two
friends meeting in a café as with the practice of a method of
treatment. To make an analogy: if I were to describe, from experience, the kind of interchange that represented a successful or
unsuccessful marriage, I would find it difficult to select a 'session'
which was either typical or crucial or presented a method, but I
could hope to give the reader an idea of the general tenor of the
relationship and provide information from which he and I may draw
some conclusion, however tenuous. I think there is a sense in which
one might say: 'I tried to make the marriage work.' But it is harder
to justify presenting a vignette from the marriage relationship in
order to say: 'Here is an example of my trying.' And even more
problematic to say: 'See me trying. If you do as I do, you too can
make your marriage work!'

This is especially true of the account which follows, for, looking
back on it after three years, I am not particularly proud of my
response and would certainly not present it as an example of excellence. However, it was probably good enough, for what I shall
describe is a typical session – selected arbitrarily in so far as this is

possible – of a therapeutic relationship which both the patient and I believed to be enriching.

What I am about to submit to the reader is, therefore, a success story – albeit a success that is modest rather than spectacular. In so doing I am not, of course, exceptional, for success is what psychotherapists write about. The reason for their preoccupation with success is not simply a narcissistic one, although it is hard to overestimate this factor. The reluctance to relate failure derives also from the pain which such an account might bring to the patient who might read it and from the fact that inept behaviour is not usually very instructive. As Simone Weil put it: 'No one is very interested if we add 2 and 2 and make 5.'

To my mind, however, the problem is less a matter of selecting therapeutic endeavours with a successful outcome (one can at least be open about this) than presenting an account which, either blatantly or subtly, distorts the facts in order to show the therapist in a good light. As this deception is largely made unconsciously I cannot hope to avoid it, but there is a certain safeguard in that the behaviour which I select as that benefiting a good psychotherapist will not necessarily be considered so by the reader.

Sarah, who is 28, had been coming to me for about eighteen months before the session I am about to report. She sought therapy because she was depressed, could find no satisfying work, had lost hope in her capacity to live with another person, and, partly as a result of a previous attempt at therapy, had come to think of herself as aggressive, manipulative, and probably unhelpable.

Although, for the sake of brevity, I shall refer to, but not describe, certain themes, I intend to set down our interchanges as fully as I can, avoiding as far as possible the temptation to reduce them to what appears relevant and significant. I do this with the aim of giving the reader a flavour of the reality of our meetings and permitting him his own deductions from material that is as unorganized and undefended as I can consciously make it. (Some readers may believe that a tape-recording is better for this purpose, but my own view is that even if one appears to forget the presence of the machine in the room it still makes its own selection of the possible.)

I opened the front door to Sarah and, on entering, she asked, 'How are you?'

'All right,' I replied. I followed her into the consulting room where she removed her shoulder bag before sitting down and gave me a rather embarrassed smile. 'I feel a bit uneasy,' she said. 'It's because of not seeing you for a week. How's your knee?'

'It's much the same, but I seem to get around on it O.K. I'm seeing the surgeon tomorrow.'

'Oh,' said Sarah anxiously, 'Does that mean an operation? Might you be in hospital?'

'Oh, no,' I replied. 'It's just that I decided to go to see him again. It's a year since I last did.' (I should explain here that a knee that I damaged in an accident two years ago has recently been giving trouble and on two occasions prevented my travelling to London to see Sarah.)

Sarah asked me more questions about the (non-medical) treatment I have been having for the knee and we discussed these and, in relation to them, Ivan Illich's book *Medical Nemesis* which I have lent her. Then she asked, 'Are you a hypochondriac like all doctors?'

'Unfortunately, yes. I've diagnosed everything except cancer so far.'

'Why do you think it's playing up now?'

I hesitated: 'Oh dear, it's complicated . . .'

'It's O.K. I can tell that perhaps you don't want to talk about it to me.'

I didn't follow up the 'to me'. I'm not sure whether she meant 'to a patient', or 'to someone non-medical', or whether she felt I wanted to keep it to myself. I think it was the latter. I said, 'Oh, no. It's not that. It's just that it really *is* complicated, especially if you believe, as I do, that a symptom is an aspect of your whole being.'

Sarah then went on to say: 'I thought, the other day, I don't really know you in other situations, do I? That's egocentric. I think you're just for me.'

'Well, I suppose, I don't always show you myself even here. For instance, I told you the facts about my knee, but I didn't tell you how awful I feel about it, how fed up I am with the bloody thing.' Sarah then questioned me in detail about my feelings and I answered her in detail. She then said: 'What made me think of you in a new light was when your daughter answered the door to me. I'd met your wife of course but I'd never met any others of your family. I don't know your age. I just didn't think of you having a grown-up daughter. She's beautiful, isn't she?'

I am rather ashamed to admit that at this point my vanity got the better of me. I try to be open about myself and it would have been natural for me to interject, telling Sarah my age, but I am not very ready to confess this fact unless asked directly, for people are usually surprised to find that I am older than I look. I also found myself wondering if Sarah were jealous of my daughter, as there are two different ways in which she might well be. In the first place she refers to herself as 'plain', compared with her sister whom she regards as 'beautiful'. In the second place she has said that it would have been a lot better for her as a child if 'someone like you had been around the place'.

Sarah then added: 'I suppose I saw you in a different role.'

'Yes, and a different generation.'

'Yes, but I don't think of you as a different generation. I judge people by their attitude more than their age. My friends Mr and Mrs Pierce are in their early sixties but I don't think of them as a different generation.'

After this exchange I found myself asking (and I cannot now remember by what route I came to the question): 'You worry about me, don't you?'

'Yes, I do. It's selfish. I don't want you to be ill and not see me.'

'But you seem to *expect* me not to come.'

'Yes I do. I expected you to phone last night saying your knee was bad.'

'It's surely an exaggerated expectation? It's only been bad twice. I turn up ninety-five per cent of the time, don't I?' (In retrospect, I can see a bit of unnecessary self-justification on my part here: I like to think of myself as reliable.)

'Yes, I know.'

'Well, it's some sort of insecurity, isn't it?'

'Yes, I'm the same about being liked. I've got friends who like me but I never believe it. I have to get them to reassure me all the time.' (Although I think it is true that Sarah has friends, and is liked, she is also isolated: she has no communication with her family and has told me that she feels incapable of living with anyone.)

I reminded Sarah of her insecure feelings in childhood, and the way in which she had always tried to be independent of people. I said, 'I think you're now learning to be dependent on people – especially on me – and it's causing you this anxiety.'

'Yes, I was so *afraid* in childhood. And then it turned to anger.' Sarah then described a really horrifying scene between her parents and herself in adolescence, from which the three of them appear to have never recovered. 'But I was a difficult and stubborn child,' she added, 'I seem to have been born selfish. I was thinking the other day that I want everything to revolve around me. You know, like the Earth before Galileo. And I can't believe that life can exist without me. I can't bear it. I can't imagine that everything will still be here when I'm dead.'

I *thought*, 'Neither can I'. But I *said*, 'I don't think you're born selfish. You're not selfish with me. But there *is* something. I think you're right about the pre-Galileo thing.' (Sarah is, on the whole, considerate to me. There have been one or two occasions when her compelling urge to have her own way has caused her to put undue coercive pressure on me, but she has readily retracted when she realized what she was doing, and is as relieved as I am when I manage to stand up to the coercion. I think that both Sarah and I would say that we have been fair with each other.)

'How can I alter?'

'I suppose knowing it helps.'

'I think it's being taught that helps. Someone showing me. That's what *you* do. You are not selfish with *me*. I'm different from you in this respect. If you were to say something nice to me I would blush and so on and it would make me feel big, it would alter my idea of myself. If *I* said something nice to you you'd probably be pleased but it wouldn't alter your opinion of yourself.'

'Yes, I would be pleased, but you're right, there *is* a difference. I think it's the way we've set it up. You expose your vulnerability. That's what a patient does. He says, "Here I am, this is me, this mess", and then is vulnerable to the therapist who might say, "Yes, and you're a real pig, aren't you?", whereas if the therapist can *honestly* say, "I still think you're O.K. I even like you", the patient feels his mess is accepted by another human being. With me, it's different. I haven't exposed my vulnerability to you in the same way. And also, if you say something nice about me, it's difficult for me to be sure it's really me that you're having the feeling about and not just me-in-the-helping-set-up. But actually I don't think it's *just* that.'

'No, nor do I. But about helping me. I think with me you are careful what you say. You choose words that fit, that don't harm me. You've got to know what I'm like. And I do the same with you. I choose my words carefully.'

I am disconcerted by her last sentence. This seems a long way from free-association. Surely she should be being spontaneous? 'Why do you do that?' I asked.

'Because I feel safe enough to,' she replied. 'I feel it's worth while talking to you seriously.'

I say, 'Yes, that makes sense.'

The session ended at this point. Unfortunately, although Sarah's marked pessimism about my leg derived, I believe, from neurotic anxiety, her assessment proved to be more accurate than mine. The knee became severely arthritic; the arthritis spread to other joints; I became ill and unable to work for two months. Sarah, in spite of her dependence, survived the break very well. We kept in touch with each other by letter. But during the last fortnight she became quite depressed; and when she returned she was despondent and alienated and had little hope for the future. Although never attacking me openly for having been ill she clearly had markedly negative feelings towards me, was reluctant to come to sessions and acted in ways that made me feel worried, irritated, and uncertain about her. We discussed the reasons for her feelings and actions. This state of affairs continued for about a fortnight. At the end of one session I put my arm around her and said, 'Sarah, I don't seem to know how to help you at the moment but I like you and care about you and will help you if I can.' She responded with a smile, saying, 'Thank you for saying that'. A few days later she seemed to have settled down and I will briefly describe a session which took place at this time.

Sarah came into the consulting room. 'How are you?' she asked. I told her I felt pretty good in myself but the knee was a bit disappointing. I then asked, 'Did you survive your party?' (She had, a few days earlier, been throwing a party and had felt anxious about it.)

'Oh, yes, much better than expected. I got sloshed, but in a nice way.'

'I know what you mean. It goes one way or the other, doesn't it?'

'Yes, it does. Well, I've had two vivid dreams that I'd like to tell you.'

The first dream (which I shall not describe in detail) was of a large room in an old house, with a leaking roof, a disconnected gas fire (which could perhaps leak), a fireplace that might not light and may smoke too much, a general untidiness and dirtiness, and furniture which seemed everywhere and cluttered up the place. But she felt something could be done about the room, even if it meant some hard work.

'I think the house was me,' Sarah said. 'That's how I feel about myself. And I think it's something to do with therapy.'

We came to the conclusion, after further discussion, that the dream, although expressing fears and doubts, was basically optimistic: that it represented her belief that she has now settled down to work again after the interruption and her attempt to estimate what needed to be done.

I will describe the second dream in detail.

'There was a robot which I had made, or at least was responsible for. In spite of being a robot he had feelings and was sensitive. Like humans, he could grow, and in fact, he was growing more capable of love. But, although he realized he was a robot he was not aware that this was an odd thing to be. He was rather naïve. For instance, he did some gardening, and a number of people, including me, brought chairs and sat round and watched him, as though he was an animal in a zoo. But he didn't see anything strange in this: he just assumed that this was what happened when someone did gardening. I felt ashamed in participating in this humiliating scene, and wanted to tell him the truth but I felt the truth would crush him, and that he would not be able to face the fact that he was regarded as an oddity.'

Sarah felt that she was the robot, but otherwise could not understand the dream. I thought she was right in identifying the robot as herself, for she does, in fact, regard herself as an oddity. She dislikes her body and believes herself to be unattractive, in spite of evidence to the contrary. She sympathizes very strongly with those who are regarded by society as ill-fitted, strange, unnatural, inferior, etc., and in the previous session had expressed her fury with a man who had denounced foreigners. The occasions when she has become most angry with me were when she suspected that I have a prejudice towards certain classes of people. She would explode in wrath, then catch herself and say, 'I'm sorry. I'm over-reacting, aren't I?'

Given this tendency of Sarah's to identify with those deemed odd, and her inability to find a mate with whom to share her life, and given my knowledge of her childhood experience, it was not difficult for me to see that her vision of the robot probably expressed fairly accurately how she felt as a child, and how, to a less extent, she still feels about herself.

Sarah concurred with my interpretation of the dream and said she realized that she was still desperately and irrationally hanging on to a defence which protected her from the risk of suddenly finding she was being patronized or not taken seriously.

I asked her if she felt I patronized her.

'No, you never do that. That's why I can talk to you. There's no one else I dare talk to. Oh. Yes. I sometimes talk to Mary. Perhaps I should pay her too.'

I suggested that one of the reasons why she had taken up acting as a career was that, however much feeling she put into a performance, she could always say, 'It wasn't the real me. I was only pretending', and thus avoid the trauma of not being taken seriously. Sarah made no comment on my suggestion and I thought that she felt it unimportant. She only said, 'It was a way of being listened to. My worst fear is of being overlooked, of being treated as though non-existent.'

At this point there was a sound of a piano being played. Sarah's face lit up. 'How lovely! Is it the man who owns the place?'

'Yes, he's a great music lover. He has a Steinway grand. He's a nice chap. I like to hear him play.'

'Do you play the piano?'

'Only a bit. I'm self-taught and don't play well. But I love music and I play on the piano at home sometimes. We have an upright, but it's a good one. I get very frustrated. I know what sounds I want to make – I think I have a feel for it – but my fingers won't do it. Surprisingly, even when I'm playing badly someone in the house might say "That sounds nice".'

I cannot quite recall the interchange at this point, but we concluded that my surprise was similar to that which can occur if one's being is enjoyed by another.

I said, 'I think some children never feel they bring joy; they have to work for it all the time and you are like that; so you had to be a robot.'

Sarah agreed. Then she noticed a copper ring on my ankle. 'I see you've tried a copper ring for your joints.'

'I try everything.'

'I saw one in a shop and wondered whether to bring one for you.'

'That was a kind thought.'

It was now the end of the session and Sarah got up to go. She said, 'I saw in the shop down the road there's a new paperback of Pablo

Neruda's poems.' I had recently lent her a different book of his poems. 'I must buy a copy and then you can borrow it. I think he's marvellous. I really get something out of them. I'll bring the book back next time.'

'I'm glad you liked the poems. I thought you might.'

After that time our relationship remained rather similar and if I were to report a later session it would not be very different in form, except for those changes in nuance when people have come to know each other better. Sarah felt happier, was able to do work more creatively, was less dependent on me, came less often, and we began to consider the end of therapy. During the course of that year the nature of her childhood neurosis had become clearer. It would seem that at some point in her early life those around her had failed to listen to something that was, for her, of vital importance to communicate – in broad terms, the expression of herself – and the only position left open to her was to maintain a pretence that left her feeling defeated and ashamed. This situation was depicted in one of her dreams.

'I had been charged by the police for some crime but was innocent. No one listened to me. My father came to court with me. He was sympathetic but did not seem surprised that I had been charged, nor was he angry with the police. It was made clear to me that if I confessed I would not be punished. In the end, feeling quite hopeless, I confessed, even though I had done nothing wrong. Then I felt ashamed of my weakness.'

Sarah had never forgiven herself for the original defeat and it seemed that, time after time throughout her life, she had unconsciously attempted to organize a situation in which she was again condemned and alone, in the hope that, with a new chance, she could win the fight to save her integrity. This manoeuvre had contributed to the periods in therapy in which she appeared to thwart my attempts to help her despite her conscious desire to get well.

On reviewing the therapeutic endeavour I think that Sarah is quite correct to lay emphasis on my capacity to hear her (as she put it). When she said, 'I wish there had been somebody like you around when I was a child,' she meant, 'Someone who would listen to me, whose presence would have avoided the traumatic experience of being in a minority-of-one.' But it is significant, I think, that I listened to her before I had appreciated (at least consciously) her childhood predicament and subsequent desperate need for a hearer. That is to say, my receptive attitude was not a consequence of careful elucidation and interpretation. To what extent my intellectual understanding of her neurosis and my communication of this understanding was crucial to the therapy is difficult to estimate accurately. But the evidence of my work with Sarah confirms my suggestion, made in the last chapter, that interpretation of the transference is not necessarily the dominant theme in a successful piece of therapy.

Readers may disagree with my interpretation of the dreams reported and I think it likely that some psychoanalysts would feel I left far too much 'material' untouched, that, for instance, I did not explore the symbolic meaning of the gas pipe, the fireplace, the furniture, and the dirt in the first dream. Yet, in spite of this thought, I feel more comfortable in describing the dreams than other areas of the sessions. The reporting of dreams is part of a widespread convention in psychotherapeutic circles; they arouse interest and can be the subject of endless and often creative exploration and speculation. And they are objective facts about a session in that they were not obviously a response to any immediate suggestion or provocation on my part. (I have never asked Sarah for dreams nor shown more interest in them than in anything else she might tell me.) My discomfort in reporting those themes (e.g. about music or poetry) which do not fit into the traditional pattern of 'psychoanalytic work' is, in part at least, a measure of the pressure that is brought to bear on a psychotherapist to behave and report and believe as efficacious certain well-established, acceptable areas of experience, and to dismiss other areas as harmful, superfluous, or of secondary importance. My impression is that the significant interchange between Sarah and myself in this session, as in most others, centres on her trust that I will not patronize her or treat her as odd: in short, that I will listen to her and respond to her with seriousness and respect. And I do this primarily from my intuition that this is what she needs and from a (less definable) desire to talk in a certain way (a way that incidentally warms and encourages her) with a person whom I do in fact like and respect, and who does not provoke me into a detrimental falseness or superficiality. If she did – as some of my patients do – then I would have to confront her with this unpleasant fact and search within myself for ways of relating to her that would be the least destructive that I could manage.

As in daily living, when things are going well – when the fit is good

– then analysis and self-analysis fall into the background. When things are going badly something needs to be done to improve the relationship. This will include the investigation of destructive factors on both sides. But we should, I believe, try to avoid the danger of becoming *preoccupied* with such a pursuit. Let me try to illustrate this point.

One feature of this report of my relationship with Sarah – which may have impressed itself on the reader – is Sarah's consideration for me. She likes to talk to me about myself, and is concerned about my well-being. I have been taught, by Freud, to suspect the motive behind such a show of interest – and with justification. In her day-to-day life Sarah shows a pattern of behaviour in which she tries hard to accommodate to the needs of others, often at her own expense, but cannot keep up this effort and has periodical explosions with highly unpleasant consequences. Inevitably we have wondered whether the same kind of thing is happening in relation to me. Is Sarah repressing hostility which then reveals itself in the 'reaction-formation' of compulsive adaptability?

On one occasion she made a comment which is relevant to the question. 'Last week, when you changed the session to the evening I wondered if I would be able to get here in time and thought of saying "Could you make it half an hour later?" But then you might have felt obliged to stay on although it was inconvenient, so I didn't ask. But perhaps I should have done.'

I do not know the answer to this question. It seems to depend on one's philosophy of living rather than a diagnosis of psychopathology. Although there were times when Sarah treated me with undue respect (an attitude which I sometimes challenged), I feel it would be doctrinaire of me – and out of keeping with my intuition – to assume that she concealed a hate of me which she would have to express in order to overcome the ambivalence with which she grew up. And I am supported in this thought by the fact that she has gradually become more able to contend with these feelings in the outer world without their appearance in *striking* form in the therapeutic set-up. We are here faced again with the question raised in the previous chapter. Should the therapist conduct himself in such a way that the patient re-experiences the traumas of childhood in the hope that they can be faced again and overcome in the therapeutic situation, or should he relate to his patient in the way he feels intuitively will be untraumatic and comforting? Sarah herself would, if asked this question, come down in favour of the latter. In attempting to describe what had helped her, she once said: 'It is the way you are to me. Right from the start I felt you treated me as an equal, that you tried to be fair with me; I didn't feel you wanted to have power over me. You don't seem to have preconceived ideas about me, putting a label on me, you've waited to let me be myself and to see what I'm like and yet you've not been distant. I've got to know you.'

I believe that Sarah is reasonably correct in her estimate. But in accepting her view one should be aware of certain possible errors.

Firstly, there is the question of authenticity. Not only is it difficult for me to convey the subtle difference between a true and a false experience, but it is also very difficult for Sarah and me to know the nature of our relationship. Are we really open to each other or are we engaged in a collusive belief, a mutual exercise in narcissism, a *folie à deux*? I have, in my life, had many relationships – with relatives, friends, colleagues, and patients – which seemed to me to be authentic but which did not stand the test of time, and I am surely not alone in this. But, unless we become entirely cynical, we continue to believe that authentic relationships can come our way and that we can know when they do so. Moreover, my relationship with Sarah *did* stand the test of time. When Sarah finally left me to marry and live in Ireland we both felt we were losing a good friend.

Secondly, it is hard to be sure that Sarah is right in her assumption that my receptive attitude has been crucial to her experience of growth. Psychotherapists – and to some extent their patients – tend to attribute the cause of improvement according to their theoretical tenets.

Thirdly, even if I am correct in my estimation of what has occurred, a false impression of the *reasons* for the occurrence may easily be given or taken. I would say that what happened was (to put it according to different philosophies of living) a matter of grace or luck. Sarah and I were suited to each other: I was able to give what she required and she helped me to give it. If she or I had been less well matched, or, in our different ways, more psychologically crippled, the outcome may have been futile. I have spent time with patients to whom I could not be receptive because I am the person that I am and cannot will myself to be other. We can place ourselves in as favourable a position as possible – by allotting sufficient time, having a quiet room, and exposing ourselves and our work to the constructive criticism of others, We can – and this is my justification for writing the present book – try to prevent the suppression, by mistaken theories, of whatever is in us to give spontaneous help. But we can do all this and still fail.

The word 'spontaneous' can readily be misleading. I do not mean to suggest an unthinking, precipitate response. Sarah herself said, in the session I have reported: 'You choose your words carefully . . . And I do the same with you.' This carefulness needs to be contrasted with inhibition. Both occurred in our relationship, but to the extent that our caution derived more from a concern not to confuse or harm each other rather than a cowardly avoidance of necessary confrontation I would say that we were spontaneous with each other. When I discussed this question with Sarah she said, 'No, I don't think we collude in that way. When I've behaved shittily to you, you've said so.' Her reply, although no guarantee, gives me some reassurance. But I think I gain more confidence from my recognition that when I am with her I do not feel the strain that comes from a need to conceal myself – a strain with which, unhappily, I am familiar when with more people than I would like to mention.

Sarah emphasizes my ordinary, non-technical approach to her and makes no reference to any specialized ability, derived from Freud or other thinkers, to interpret her symptoms or dreams. It is clearly the former that has the greatest impact on her. She could be saying two rather different things:

1. 'Out of all the ways you are towards me, technical or non-technical, I select the latter as the most helpful ones', or

2. 'The way you are towards me is primarily non-technical and it is because of this primacy that you can help me.'

Having not questioned her on this point I am not sure which she means, but I would suggest that, although both statements have some validity, the second is probably nearer the truth since it approximates to the way I believe myself to have been with her.

If, indeed, Sarah is correct, then she is saying that this is the way I – a particular person, a particular therapist – am able to help. It is likely that other therapists help their patients in other ways: one could, for example, imagine a therapist who relied entirely on the interpretation of non-verbal behaviour and who made no attempt to contact the patient in an ordinary way. Presumably any assessment his patient might make of the nature of the help received would be notably different from that made by Sarah.

I am inclined to agree with Sarah's assessment because I believe that it is chiefly by means of my personal approach to people that I help them, that the success or failure of therapy depends on whether I have *this* rather than *that* attitude towards them. But I am still left with the question: 'Have I found a mode of working that is suitable for *me* but not necessarily for other therapists?'

Every approach to another human being is personal in the sense that it affects a part of him which is tuned towards the whole relationship between two people. If I engage a patient with the belief that what is important is, say, to interpret his dreams, massage his body, or desensitize him from a fear of groups, then in the pursuit of this aim I will, if I am rigorous, orientate our relationship to this end, and am bound to adopt a different (more technical) attitude to him than I took towards Sarah. But I believe that a price would be exacted for this stance. My focus would, to an extent, diminish my chances of providing a medium in which the other person may explore his possibilities for growth in flexible conditions.

It would appear that, in aiming to help a patient, one is left with the choice of a general or particular approach. The general approach is ordinary in the sense that it has much in common with encounters between friends in everyday living and is special only in the intensity and rigour of its focus on facilitating the growth of the other in a somewhat unusual set-up; the particular puts its trust in a specific aim and/or method (e.g. abreaction, negative conditioning) with the implicit assumption that this approach is of such paramount importance that any limitation it may of necessity bring to the personal encounter is, even if regrettable, a price worth paying. Therapists who put their faith in the particular usually do all they can to overcome the ways in which their technique gets in the way of an ordinary relationship: they develop interest in their patients as people, encourage them to fullness, openness, intimacy, and often grow fond of them – but when this occurs it is *in spite of* the technique. One cannot have one's cake and eat it. Whether the personal approach is one that is suitable for some therapists and not others, or whether it is a desirable aim for all who seek to help those psychologically disturbed, remains open to debate. I write this book with the latter belief, setting down some of my own experiences in the hope that they carry conviction, and putting forward arguments to support the general application of this experience.

Therapists come in all sorts of shapes and sizes, with different styles of living, different philosophies, different neuroses and inhibitions and counter-inhibitions: they can be sceptical or gullible, dull or exciting, gentle or aggressive, forthcoming or reticent, and so on. Their way of being with the patient will be modified, but not eliminated, by their theoretical conception of the nature of psychotherapy. They will usually be sufficiently flexible to adapt their styles, at least to some extent, according to the needs of their patients. What I wish to single out is the attitude – which, for want of a better term I shall call 'receptive' – that seemed of value in my attempt to help Sarah. It is an attitude which is exploratory in a way that aims to permit the other person to reveal himself, in his own manner and in his own time, with the minimum of coercive pressure from outside, and without the assumption that he can be neatly fitted into one's own system of thought.

The attitude of mind that I am suggesting as a first approach to a therapeutic endeavour is one which, at least provisionally, gives the other person the benefit of the doubt. Freud's advice was that psychoanalysis should be undertaken in a spirit of 'benevolent scepticism' – a characteristically accurate phrase for his approach and those who have followed him. It is an attitude which, I believe, derived not only from his identification with the natural scientist but from a determination to avoid painful and humiliating seduction (in the general sense) by his patients. It ensures that certain mistakes will not be made. But it is slightly different from the attitude which, first and foremost, allows the other person to be and become in a facilitating setting. In the latter case the therapist will be less alerted to making a criticism (to being 'sceptical', in however 'benevolent' a way); he will be less the detached observer than the listener who identifies with the other's experience, becomes involved with the drama, and thereby risks the possibility of naïvety. But this is still not quite like an ordinary relationship, for the patient is seeking help and it is incumbent upon the therapist to remember this: to place his own needs in the background, to listen, wonder, and reflect. To say to the person, as it were, 'You have given me quite a task here. Forgive me if sometimes I pause and think more than might seem natural to you, if I forego (and cause you to forego) some of the richness that might occur if I did not have this task.' The difference, I think, is one of emphasis. Whereas the attitude of 'benevolent scepticism' places the task (of criticism) at the centre of the stage, the attitude I am suggesting focuses on an attempt to understand the other primarily by experiencing his presence, by living with him for a while in a situation gauged towards receiving what he is. (In noting that this endeavour – psychotherapy – is to be distinguished from other relationships in ordinary life I do not want to exaggerate this difference. In ordinary living, in any fruitful and intimate relationship, it is incumbent upon the two people to listen, sometimes to reflect, and sometimes to criticize. The characteristic of psychotherapy is that the onus to behave in this way is more – but by no means entirely – on one of the two people.)

A recognition of the importance of receptivity in therapy should not be taken to imply that, for example, it is necessarily wrong to expound one's own view of life to a patient, or to shout at him or control him, but I do believe that if these were one's characteristic ways of relating to a person in therapy, then one would be better occupied elsewhere. This line of thought leads me to the conclusion that an attitude of receptivity is a quality which, although not confined to psychotherapists, nor the only quality that psychotherapists should be expected to manifest, is perhaps an attitude which more than any other brings the possibility of successful therapeutic action. If, by contrast, a therapist's actions are characterized by direction, dominance, or impingement, then his work is so far removed from that which I understand by psychotherapy then he is in a different business from mine and his approach is not the subject of this book.*

I stand by this view because it is the way I find I can best work. In so doing I feel myself part of a movement which, from Freud onwards, places receptivity at the centre of its *practice*, although not at the centre of its *theory*. Indeed, those writers – notably Jung, Boss, and Winnicott – who openly acknowledge the immense importance of receptivity are in the minority. Rather, I would say that psychotherapy, even that within the tradition I espouse, is generally assumed to depend more on the capacity to *do something to the patient*.

Although I realize that there are factors in my own life which

* For this reason I often feel myself close to those in other disciplines from mine who try to ensure that their insights and theories do not impinge unduly on those with whom they work. I think, for example, of David Holbrook's sensitive discussion of the dangers of interpreting the symbolism of children's creative writing – see Holbrook, D. (1973), *English in Australia Now*, Cambridge University Press, London, pp. 176 ff.

have led me to identify readily with those whose lives have been crippled by the impingement of others, and to wish to offer them a second chance of growth with the minimum of coercion, I do not feel alone in this respect. Is it not likely that the majority of those who have been drawn to the field of psychotherapy and have found that they can work adequately in it have done so for reasons not dissimilar from mine, that those of us who are in the right job have an intuitive recognition of the need to be receptive? Receptivity is a complex response, and may at times involve the therapist in behaving in ways such as fooling around, being angry, revealing his gifts and deficiencies and inner feelings, and so on; and therefore the arguments in its favour coincide in many ways with the arguments that can be adduced to justify a 'personal' response. For this reason I was interested to note that David Smail, in his recent book *Psychotherapy: A Personal Approach*, makes frequent use of the word 'encouragement' in contexts in which I would probably write 'receptivity' – but I believe we have in mind the same kind of thing.

The therapist who sees his role as purely technical is likely to approach his patients with a kind of psychological tool-kit which, once he has exhausted its capabilities without success, will leave him despairingly bereft of ideas. On the other hand, the therapist who sees his 'technical' activity as flexibly in the service of the general aim of encouragement, will be able to adapt his strategies to the unique set of meanings generated in the relationship between himself and his patient – and he will be able to make new tools, without for example, worrying about whether they conform to specifications established by the 'laws of behavioural science'. As long as they fit in with the patient's personal set of meanings, as long as *he* can use them, they will fill the bill quite adequately.[1]

I do not quite agree with Smail's way of putting this but I admire his book and find it encouraging (to use his word) that someone coming from such a different intellectual background from mine (behaviour therapy as opposed to psychoanalysis) has struggled to a stance rather similar to my own.

We do not have to look hard to find other areas in life in which the receptive attempt to help another to grow is neglected and corrupted by overzealous impingement. Education immediately springs to mind. But I would like to end this chapter with a brief reference to the failure of society to receive a parturient mother and her baby in an appropriate manner, for it would seem that the function of a midwife and that of a psychotherapist are in some ways similar.

A number of years ago I took part in a study of mothers suffering from severe 'post-partum depression' and came to recognize that, among the many factors which contributed to their states of mind, one was the experience of hospital confinement. Pursuing this line of thought further I concluded that the attitude of Western society to childbirth is dangerously intrusive.[2] A recently published symposium, *The Place of Birth*, gives ample support to my fears. The suffering of mothers who wish to take responsibiltiy for their own births, the obstacles put in their way, and the determination of some of them to avoid intrusiveness is striking. Sheila Kitzinger writes:

Many obstetricians did not take women's fears, or their reasons for preferring a home confinement, very seriously. In discussion with her consultant, a woman said that she wanted to avoid Pethidine because of the possible deleterious effect on the baby, and that she felt that she might reduce the need for drugs if she had a home birth. He said, jokingly, that Pethidine must be acceptable as he had it when he was born, and if the current thinking that it impaired development was right, then he would have been an absolute genius, instead of an ordinary genius. When I pressed him further about home confinements, and about some people's fear of being in a strange institution, he asked me if I would want to die at home, seeing I was so keen on giving birth at home. He was genuinely surprised that I said, 'Yes, I would like to die at home, surrounded by loved ones.' And she concluded: 'I think it worrying that these men have so much control over birth, and yet seem to understand so little about life.'[3]

Another contributor to the symposium, Lewis Mehl, assesses 'The Outcome of Home Delivery Research in the United States'. In a section about the 'home delivery attendants', he writes:

The attitudes and philosophies of these practitioners towards birth and towards the indications for obstetrical intervention were remarkably similar from group to group and were very different from hospital practitioners. Uniformly the home practitioners' criteria for indications for intervention were more rigorous and exclusive than the hospital practitioners'. Interventions were made less often by the home practitioners and unusual labours classified more frequently as normal variants by the home practitioners than by the hospital practitioners. Clearly the hospital practitioners believed that their aggressive technological approach improved outcomes, whereas the home delivery practitioners believed that much of this was unnecessary and occasionally even dangerous.[4]

I make this comparison because I believe we are faced with a pervasive distortion in our society of which obstetrics and psychotherapy are but two examples. An impersonal method intrudes upon the individual to a degree that many of us find unacceptable, and, in the face of this assault, the need for receptivity is forgotten. This fact is blatant in the field of general psychiatry. In psychotherapy it is more subtly evident: it reveals itself in an over-readiness to make interpretations, a too easy reliance on special theory, a nervous desire for 'scientific' validation of treatment, a preoccupation with qualification of students at the expense of teaching, and the increasing influence of 'behaviour modification' techniques.

I will try, in sum, to put the thesis of this chapter as briefly as possible. If I am to help another I am unlikely to be successful unless I first have reverence for his being and his growth, and give due recognition to this reverence in my theory. In the field of psychotherapeutics irreverence takes the form of undue impingement by means of intrusive 'interpretations' or 'behaviour modification'.

What I state is a belief which one either holds or does not. I am not advocating from a moral point of view that we try to be nice and tolerant and receptive to our patients. Rather, I am suggesting that our society idealizes impingement, and the resulting failure to put receptivity at the centre of our conception of our work is *incorrect* in that it underrates the capacity of most people to grow if given sufficient time in relatively favourable conditions.

References

1. Lomas, P. (1966), 'Ritualistic Elements in the Management of Childbirth', *Brit. J. Med. Psychol.* 39. 207.
2. Kitzinger, S. and Davis, J. (eds.), *The Place of Birth,* Oxford University Press, Oxford.
3. Kitzinger, S. (1978), 'Women's Experience of Birth at Home', in *The Place of Birth*, ed. Kitzinger, S. and Davis, J., Oxford University Press, Oxford.
4. Mehl, L. (1978), 'The Outcome of Home Delivery Research in the United States', in *The Place of Birth*, ed. Kitzinger, S. and Davis, J., Oxford University Press, Oxford.

6. Criticism

'No one else with any suggestions? Well, for your
preparation, let me have a translation of the whole passage
and see what you can make of it. Try to keep as close to the
text as you can but without obscuring the real meaning.'
    The real meaning? How in a phrase can one express the
real meaning of one's whole life, of the whole world?
Drusilla, after all, was only 15 and Miss Wace was 55 and
had had 40 more years in which to grow the protective
camouflage of her sharp inquisitive humour, the leathery
time-chiselled skin, the stab and plunge of the tortoiseshell
hairpins. – Esme Dodderidge, *The Lesson*

The suggestion I made in the last chapter that receptivity is a crucial
element in the practice of psychotherapy and is endangered by our
current preoccupation with intrusive procedures does not con-
travene the fact that people do – and must – impinge upon each
other. Mutual criticism forms part of any healthy relationship.
Provided that it is informed – that it derives from a receptive
understanding of the other – and is neither based upon destructive
or defensive aims nor is the outcome of a misguided philosophy, it
can bring enlightenment. Someone who comes for help may not
openly say 'Please criticize me', but such a request is implied in his
coming. If he feels confused and lost, if his life is crippled or in ruins,
he will surely hope that the therapist will be able to say something
about the ways in which he has erred and the beliefs that have led to
his undoing.
    In ordinary life we need, and justifiably offer, criticisms of each
other's blind spots, in a way that is not unlike the critique that
occurs in psychoanalysis. I cannot improve on Schafer's wording of
this point. He considers that:

. . . any thoughtful person generally accepts the idea that we do not observe
or know ourselves accurately in every respect. This is so as much for how we
remember our personal histories as it is for how we view our present
temperaments and our behaviour in relationships with others. Moreover,
we are especially likely to observe ourselves inaccurately in those areas of
life where we feel more emotionally aroused or conflicted – say, ashamed,
guilty, envious, enamoured or enraged. A corollary of this point is that we
do not observe other people accurately in every respect either. Again, this
is especially likely to be the case when our strongest and most conflictual
emotions are aroused.

Accepting that people are unreliable reporters of their past and present lives, one does not hesitate, in daily life, to disagree with them in these connections. That is to say, one allows oneself to declare that one knows them better than they know themselves. On their part, of course, others may do the same to us, and perhaps with equally good warrant. We do learn about ourselves from others; common sense in human relationships requires us to accept the idea that we develop and maintain blind spots. By blind spots I mean not only that a person may be unaware of major aspects of how he or she behaves in the world; I mean, also, that a person may be insistently oblivious or uncomprehending in this respect. In accepting the idea of blind spots, we are accepting the idea that significant features of people's lives may be dominated by unconscious tendencies or characteristics, and that perhaps only an independent observer might be able to recognise the fact. But we go farther than this, for on many occasions we even presume to interpret the meaning of some of these blind spots; that is to say, we may infer that they are ways of protecting one's vanity or denying one's guilt feelings, or that they are excesses characteristic of the rapture of love or the bitterness of hate. In making these interpretations, we are treating the blind spots as intelligible on the assumption that they are unconsciously motivated.[1]

In some relationships criticism does not assume a central position. A person may ask me what I think about his behaviour and whether I can throw light on the reason for it; sometimes we discuss (and occasionally disagree about) how life should be lived; and sometimes we scrutinize how we are, or should be, with each other. But, on the other hand, criticism may dominate the interchange. It may, for instance, be either demanded or avoided like the plague. In the former case – assuming that the desire is not a masochistic one – the therapist is called upon to offer a challenge, a stimulating critique, for which the other person senses a need and feels strong enough to weather, trusting that he will be judged with understanding and compassion. By contrast, in the latter case the patient may lack the capacity to face the discomforting truths which are bound to arise in any rigorous mutual exploration and the therapist may be left with no choice other than a considered – and possibly even traumatic – impingement of the other's self-determination. Such a criticism is a composed equivalent of the violent action which may be taken in extreme situations, as, for instance, when a patient advances upon an open window with the intention of hurling himself out of it.

It may be useful to differentiate between a critique which

emerges out of a mutual exploration and which is basically conso-
nant with the person's presentation of himself, and one which flies
in the face of this presentation. Psychoanalysis, because of its origins
and the dramatic nature of its early insights, has erred in its preoccupation with the latter. It appeals to the magician in us, to the child
who delights in having something special up his sleeve with which to
impress, surprise, and disconcert. It has – or once had – shock
value. To say this is not to discount the insights but to suggest that
they have tended to an unjustified arrogance which, by overestimat-
ing the need for and use of dissonant criticism (that is, criticism that
does not simply flow from the person's immediate over-all experience of himself in a receptive setting), can easily interfere with a
true understanding of the other.

It might be thought that I am merely concerned with different
styles of being: gentle or rough, cautious or adventurous. To some
extent – but only to some extent – I am. There is, I believe, in the
psychotherapeutic world, a taboo on gentleness (comparable perhaps to the taboo on tenderness so well described by Suttie[2]) which
probably has deep roots but which, superficially, derives from an
idealization of the 'hard facts' of science and the stark confrontation
designed to unmask concealed aggression in therapeutic encounters. 'Let there be no sloppy sentimentality', proclaims this school
of thought; 'We are rigorous and give no quarter to such old-
fashioned values as delicacy and tact'. My doubts about the value of
this kind of attitude primarily concern the concept of continuity.

When someone seeks our help it would seem useful to try to
understand him in the context of his own experience, with due
reverence for the person that he is and believes himself to be.
Perhaps during the course of the exploration we find the need to
confront him with a startling new experience, quite disconnected
from his own previous knowledge. But to base our work on this kind
of formula is less psychotherapy (as I understand the word) than a
kind of religious or philosophical conversion. The emphasis which
psychoanalysis places on such interventions is perhaps the reason
why, however unjustly, it is sometimes condemned as a brain-
washing technique. The practitioner who is orientated to continuity, and circumspect about imposing dogma, will nevertheless, if
he hopes to promote growth, be open to the unknown and aware of
the surprising revelations of those who have previously explored his
field of work; but if in the course of his research he seizes upon an

insight that is, at least for him, of great moment, he may become more of a prophet and less of a therapist.

It would seem that a psychotherapist (and, indeed, anyone concerned to preserve the true being of the other) is in a delicately balanced position between tradition and a critique of tradition. Those who turn to him for help do not necessarily seek a prophet but, in view of the fact that their problems have developed within and, in a sense, have been engendered by a certain society, it is important that the therapist be able to criticize the milieu sufficiently well to understand its contribution to that person's downfall. If, for example, a woman suffers from an incapacitating envy of men as a consequence of growing up in a male-centred society, she will gain little help from a therapist who is not himself free from sexual prejudice.

To put the matter another way: psychotherapy is (or should be) a practice which encourages a person to act by his own agency rather than submit unthinkingly to the will of another. This is incorporated in the philosophy of living expressed by practitioners – such as Erich Fromm, Rollo May, and Abraham Maslow – who, following Paul Tillich, emphasize the 'courage to be'. Those of us who take this stance will necessarily be careful lest our own interventions endanger the autonomy of the other and should therefore look closely at the bases of our critique of the patient. What are they?

Firstly, criticism may be made of inconsistencies. It is not immediately obvious that inconsistency is wrong. A case could be made out for considering an even tenor of living to be a manifestation of dullness, and there certainly exist those who take delight in presenting themselves as unpredictable, muddle-headed, or gnomic. But most of us recognize that a measure of integration is necessary if we are to be taken seriously by others, and will be upset if we are shown to be inconsistent. I will give a simple example, of a kind that will be very familiar to practising therapists.

Some years ago a young student came to see me because of a severe word block. This man treated me with a formality and deference that was almost unctuous, denied that he had any negative feelings (such as anger, contempt, competitiveness, or envy) towards me, and appeared well satisfied to keep this distance between us. Yet in his dreams we rolled together on the floor in drunken orgies. One day a copy of an article written by me fell into his hands and his behaviour towards it was quite striking. Despite

an expressed interest in its contents he could not, for one reason or
another, manage to look at it, telling me he couldn't find the time,
and that his wife didn't like him to read in the house, albeit that, in
fact, he read profusely at home. Finally he lost the article. These
examples give some idea of the discrepancies between his professed
and his concealed attitudes to me. Disparities of this kind form the
basis of the mammoth work of Janet, Freud, and Jung, and are the
major focus of contemporary psychoanalysis.*

Secondly, the therapist may criticize the behaviour of the patient
from a simple, naïve, subjective point of view, conveying in effect,
'I don't like what you do'. He may, for example, say, 'You bore me
to death', 'Why do you always moan?', 'When I'm with you I feel
pinned down and inhibited, and want to get away. What are you
doing to make me feel that way?', and so on.

The utility of such criticisms lies in the fact that the patient has
come to someone who is prepared to be open and truthful, for the
sake of greater understanding, even at the risk of hurt and disharmony. The setting increases the chance that the patient will take the
criticism as a genuine attempt to help rather than a sadistic or
retaliatory attack. Its validity rests entirely on the capacity of one
human being – the therapist – to respond without too much distortion to the patient's behaviour. The response may be made quickly,
spontaneously, and emotionally, or, after reflection, in a considered, measured way.

Thirdly, the therapist may criticize his patient from the basis of a
general philosophy of living. For instance: 'Why do you hold yourself aloof from people? Surely love and intimacy add to the richness
of life? Can you afford to ignore them?', or, 'I notice that you
always avoid risk. But a full life involves risk, and it seems to me
that you are impoverishing yourself.'

It is not easy for a therapist to justify this kind of criticism. He is
not an oracle and has no reason to set himself up as knowing better

---

* David Ingleby has recently argued[3] that psychoanalysis, although deriving its
force from a critique of common sense, is itself grounded in common sense. 'This is
only possible if common sense contains *contradictions* – so that the exposure of
contradictions in the realm of the "obvious" must be the essence of any "depth
hermeneutics".

This, in fact, is an apt description of Freud's whole project. Unlike both the
positivist and the mystic – who claim privileged access to a transcendent plane of
"reality", from which common sense appears as an out and out delusion – the
psychoanalyst starts from the same criteria for interpretation as anybody else . . .'

than his fellows how one should live. Yet he is bound, if only implicitly, to make judgements. The danger of harm to the patient from such action can be lessened by humility on the part of the therapist and alertness on the part of the patient. The latter's vulnerability is great: he can only hope that – and try to assess whether – he has entrusted himself to someone with a valuable approach to living. The therapist is of course also in danger of malign influence, but because he is not – at least in this set-up – primarily turning to another to guide him through unknown territory, his vulnerability is less.

How is a critique of a person best made? This is one of the questions that has engendered the present book. Our way of being is, in a sense, a critique of others. If I behave in an admirable way – if, say, I am courageous – I not only set an example to others but I make an implicit critique. Is it possible that this kind of critique is the most convincing? We might say, of another's action, 'You are a coward', but our statement may carry less weight than if we were to show courage in our dealings with him. If this is the case – if our actions speak louder than our words – we need to seriously consider its bearing on the practice of psychotherapy. To accept this suggestion does not, of course, exclude an intellectual critique of the other person, but may lessen the enthusiasm which we, in a scientific age, place upon such an approach.

In considering the effect on the patient of our behaviour, we have to beware of becoming too self-conscious about what we do. In psychoanalytical writings the idea is frequently put forward that the analyst offers himself as a model for 'identification', that because of the method of treatment the patient regresses to a childlike attitude towards the analyst and 'introjects' the good qualities of the latter. This is a perfectly legitimate description of the process, but, put in this way, it tempts the therapist towards a cautious, if not narcissistic, attitude of correct behaviour, characteristic of moral leaders from school prefects to archbishops. Furthermore, the theory of identification with the analyst becomes so well known that many educated people – particularly those who work within the psychotherapeutic field – have to struggle not only with the authentic conflict over excessive identification during therapy but with the widespread supposition that this is bound to occur. It is one thing – and useful – to note the danger of over-identification; it is another to be tormented by the assumption that it will occur to a dangerous degree. In this way theory polarizes the conflict. If, however, we stay – as I believe we should when possible – with the ordinary way of putting things, we will more readily see that the flow of influence is *two way*, and we will therefore be able to act and speak with greater freedom of expression. A straightforward, simple criticism between equals is a very different matter from that made by a person who appears to possess a superior framework of thought. (I have already discussed this danger (Chapter 4) in relation to transference interpretations in which the therapist claims that the patient's perception of him is a mere distortion derived from past experience.)

The issue of criticism has, I think, been obscured in psychoanalytical thinking because of the failure to recognize that 'interpretation' – the basis of Freud's work – is not a simple matter of rectifying perceptual error and replacing it with objective truth but may involve a difference of opinion in which no overview is available.

That Freud's theoretical edifice rests on the capacity of the therapist to understand, interpret, or elucidate that which is unknown or obscure to the patient should not surprise us. His endeavour took place at a time when scientific explanation was already accepted by most thinkers as the most appropriate approach to the physical and biological world, and efforts were already being made to account for human behaviour in similar terms. In the light of this philosophy it would seem an obvious thing to do to approach a person in distress by asking: 'Why is he like this? Let us look beneath the surface of this phenomenon into the underlying factors and causes. Let us interpret what is manifest in terms of its hidden structure and meaning.' There is nothing essentially wrong in doing this. It helped Freud towards important insights into individual experience, just as it has helped Lévi-Strauss, Chomsky, and Goffman to insights in other areas of human experience.

Rycroft defines interpretation as:

The process of elucidating and expounding the meaning of something abstruse, obscure, etc. Psychoanalytical interpretations are statements made by the analyst to the patient in which he attributes to a dream, a symptom, or a chain of free associations some meaning over and above (under and below) that given to it by the patient. The paradigm of interpretation is dream-interpretation, the activity of discovering the latent content of meaning of a dream by analysis of its manifest content.[4]

Elsewhere Rycroft elaborates this definition into a conception of psychoanalysis that is illuminating:

If psychoanalysis is recognised as a semantic theory not a causal one, its theory can start where its practice does – in the consulting-room, where a patient who is suffering from something in himself which he does not understand confronts an analyst with some knowledge of the unconscious – i.e. who knows something of the way in which repudiated wishes, thoughts, dreams, and who knows, as it were, the grammar and syntax of such translations and is therefore in a position to interpret them back again into the communal language of consciousness. According to the scientific analyst this can only be done by elucidating and reconstructing the history of the illness and of its infantile origins, but even he agrees that this is useless unless the analyst has made contact (*rapport* with the patient) and it seems to me that it makes better sense to say that the analyst makes excursions into historical research in order to understand something which is interfering with his present communication with the patient (in the same way as a translator might turn to history to elucidate an obscure text) than to say that he makes contact with the patient in order to gain access to biographical data. In the former he is using the past to understand the present, in the latter he is using his biographical research to legitimise his *rapport* with the patient by formulating it in terms of a theory about the causes of neurosis.[5]

This clear statement about the nature of psychoanalysis (which applies also to all 'analytically orientated' methods) increases the urgency with which we must question the assumption that interpretation is the key, the *sine qua non*, the Royal Road of psychotherapy, and distinguish its meaning from that of criticism and understanding.

What gives one the feeling of being understood? It would seem to be a belief that the listener has an over-all, global impression of oneself, that he accepts some perceptions as tentative and provisional approximations, does not worry unduly about the unknowns and uncertainties, and is prepared to wait, recognizing that in some ways one is not only unknown but unknowable.

There is a colloquial use of the word in which this significance is central. We will say, for example: 'I apologized to Mr Brown for giving him the wrong newspaper and explained that my small son had thrown the original one on the fire. He was very understanding.' This statement implies that Mr Brown has been magnanimous about the matter: that he allowed for the vagaries of existence, knew that human beings were less than perfect, and therefore was able to be flexible and forgiving, with a result likely to be 'therapeutic' in that particular situation.

Understanding is, in this sense, a very broad term, rather akin to 'knowing'. It refers to a recognition of the totality of the other person and his situation, and implies a positive relationship in which empathy is possible. Although there appears, at first sight, to be no logical reason why we should not be able to 'understand' (in the sense of 'perceive accurately') those to whom we are indifferent or even hostile, it is commonly recognized that in actual life negative or hostile attitudes stand in the way of true perspective. And the case has been well argued philosophically by Roger Poole.[6] (The fact that 'blind love' can also distort perspective does not alter the position, for such misplaced passion stands in opposition not only to understanding but to a realistic and unselfish valuation of the other.)

My understanding of another person depends on my experience of living, and will include knowledge which will be outside the direct relationship with him. For instance, if I meet Mr Robinson, who has an obvious limp, I will conclude that his limp will have some bearing on his attitude to life, and I shall be on the alert for clues as to the nature of its effect on him – a dangerous conclusion to draw since I may lose sight of the man himself by placing him in the category of people-who-limp, but a viewpoint that I can hardly fail to adopt. I might reach this conclusion by various roads. Perhaps I empatheti- cally understand something of my own feelings were I in his posi- tion. Or I may have some disability myself. Or I may know from experience that physical disabilities have a profound effect on the victim's attitude to life. To take the matter a little further, I may, after spending a certain time with Mr Robinson, intuitively and by observation, together with logical reasoning and specialized know- ledge, acquire more direct evidence of the psychological effects of the disability and learn something of its particular place in Mr Robinson's life.

Indirect methods of enquiry, although possible to perform in the absence of any warm and intimate relationship with Mr Robinson (indeed, to some extent possible without meeting or knowing any- thing about him except for the fact that he had a limp), may lead me to a greater knowledge of him and pave the way for a closer relationship. In other words, accurate perceptions of relevant clues and an interpretation of their meaning facilitate the emergence of empathic understanding between people, but they do not by them- selves constitute such understanding, nor do they guarantee its emergence. In relation to psychotherapy the question we therefore must ask is not 'Can insights derived from a body of theoretical knowledge or method (e.g. Freudian theory, gestalt psychology, transactional analysis) be useful in understanding the other?', for the answer is simply and surely an affirmative one. But rather: 'To what extent and in what manner is such an approach helpful? Does it constitute the main *raison d'être* of psychotherapy or is it a useful but dangerous tool?'

The capacity for empathy does not preclude criticism. It is, of course, important for someone to feel that his plight is understood, that a certain predicament is seen to be what it is. For instance, if he is angry not because of childish rage against frustration but because impossible demands are being made of him then it may be vital to his sense of security and trust in the therapist that the latter is able to recognize that he is stating the truth. But what of the occasions when the patient is wrong? When he is too unlearned or afraid or confused to speak or know the truth and either withholds information or presents a false picture of the state of affairs? The need is then for the therapist to show an understanding that is, in this particular matter, beyond that of the patient, an understanding that involves criticism. He may be able to do this from his own experience of error and limitation in situations comparable to that of the patient. Or he may criticize on the basis of a knowledge of human behaviour gained from other sources, which will vary according to the degree of obscurity of the problem. If, for instance, a patient were to say, 'Yesterday I gave my boss a box of cigars because he looked unhappy', the therapist, knowing the true relationship between the patient and his boss, might say, with justification: 'Come off it, John, you know damned well you gave him the cigars because you're hoping for promotion.' This would not normally be called an interpretation, an elucidation, an application of the psychotherapeutic technique and theory but, more likely, straight talking, common sense, honesty, unsparing criticism. But suppose that the therapist were then to pursue the matter further and say: 'You have to suck up to your boss because he makes you think of your father, and you always had to suck up to your father, didn't you?' Is this an interpretation? And, in making such a comment, is the therapist departing from the method of ordinary discussion and adopting a specialized technique, thus revealing himself as a specialist of the understanding of human experience? But he may turn even more from the ordinary discourse and say, 'The cigar stands for the internalized mother's penis with which you wish to impregnate your boss/father' . . . and so on. At what point does the 'therapist' reveal himself to be an 'analyst'? I believe the answer to this question is crucial. It can only be given, however, if we have detailed knowledge of the therapist's manner, of his assumption when making this comment, and of the circumstances which led to his making it, his subsequent procedure, and the frequency with which he makes such interpretations – that is to say, his total relationship with the patient and the degree to which it is affected by an interpretative method. Let me give an example.

In the previous chapter I presented some extracts of my work with a patient – Sarah – in the hope of conveying the general tenor of our relationship, and the reader will, I expect, have noted that our conversations were closer, in content and manner, to those of ordinary living than most written examples of psychoanalytic method. One feature of the discourse was the relative lack of interpretations. But there have also been occasions in the therapy when I found myself making an interpretation in the 'classical' Freudian manner.

One day Sarah said to me: 'At the weekend I felt very low. I thought "I shan't go to Peter any more. The therapy isn't doing me any good. I still haven't got a man to love me and I never shall." I know I was being unfair. You have done me good and most times I feel better. And it didn't really seem to be about you at all.'

I said, 'It reminds me of how you turned your back in hate towards your parents. I think you want to get on with me but something in you makes you hate me for letting you down as you feel your parents let you down. There's something I don't do for you. I think you feel I don't love you enough to make you feel feminine and sexual – just as your father didn't.'

'But I believe you like me and think of me as feminine.'

'Yes, but that doesn't seem to convince you of your sexuality. I believe the only thing that would do it would be if I said, "You are the only woman in the world for me and I want to divorce Diane (my wife) and marry you instead".'

Sarah grinned. 'I believe you're right. But that would give me another kind of headache, wouldn't it?'

'Yes, as it would if your father had said it. But I think you wanted him to.'

'I can't believe *that* bit. He was awful to me. He shouted at me and he never cuddled or kissed me.'

We talked about parents and children and what was 'usual' or 'natural' behaviour between them. Then Sarah said, 'Oh God! I've just remembered a fantasy I used to have about my father. An atom bomb destroyed everybody on earth except my father and me. But the human species had to go on so he and I had to have sexual intercourse even though I didn't want it.'

This example gives some idea of my indebtedness to Freud but, taken in isolation and not in the context of my account in the previous chapter, it would give the impression that the nature of our relationship is based on a psychoanalytic model.

Few people in our society nowadays would find it difficult to entertain the possibility that a boss may represent a father. Most would take such a notion so much for granted that they would not consider it to be an interpretation of a symbol, let alone believe that such a thought might be considered an implicit acceptance of Freudian theory. With what ease such an interpretation could have been made before Freud, I am not sure. It seems obvious enough; but, as we know, it often takes genius to bring the obvious to our attention. But it would seem justified to assume that Freud has made such 'interpretations' both more possible and more likely. The difference between the man-in-the-street and the Freudian is that the latter, in view of his experience, applies the insights of Freud with greater frequency and confidence: presumably he would not require an obvious specificity of fit before interpreting a patient's behaviour in the light of certain past experiences. We are not here dealing with the question as to whether a certain Freudian therapist is, on the one hand, classical, traditional, mainstream, or rigid as opposed to one who is flexible, neo-Freudian, modern, or an adherent of a modified school of thought such as the Kleinian. Rather we are concerned with a more fundamental question as to whether the therapist sees his role to be that of someone who interprets the words of the patient in terms of a particular system of thought. To do so is the mark not only of the psychoanalyst, of whatever variety, but also of all those who seek to 'modify' the behaviour of others according to a systematic plan. If there exists a system which is clearly superior to that which we normally use in our everyday life – a system by means of which we could make a confident critique of others – then we should go straight to a teacher and learn it with all due haste. But I believe there is not.

References

1. Schafer, R. (1977), 'Psychoanalysis and Commonsense', *The Listener*, 10 November.
2. Suttie, I. (1960), *The Origins of Love and Hate*, Penguin, London.
3. Ingleby, D. (1981), 'Understanding Mental Illness', in *Critical Psychiatry*, ed. Ingleby, D., Penguin, London.
4. Rycroft, C. (1968), *A Critical Dictionary of Psychoanalysis*, Nelson, London.
5. Rycroft, C. (1966), 'Causes and Meaning', in *Psychoanalysis Observed*, ed. Rycroft, C., Constable, London, p. 18.
6. Poole, R. (1975), 'From Phenomenology to Subjective Method', *University Quarterly*, 29. 412.

7. The Language of Psychotherapy

Let us not fill our mouths
with so many faltering names,
with so many sad formalities,
with so many pompous letters,
with so much of yours and mine,
with so many signing of papers.

I have a mind to confuse things,
unite them, make them new born,
mix them up, undress them,
until all light in the world
has the oneness of the ocean,
a generous, vast wholeness,
a crackling, living fragrance. – Pablo Neruda, 'Too Many Names'

As I begin this chapter it is a bleak day in February. I sit looking out
at the wind-swept trees, and I try to think about language. I have a
sense of unease and emptiness. Then my glance falls upon a cycla-
men plant on the window-sill. I cannot describe it. A poet would
make a better job of this than I. But I am suddenly aware of the
barrenness and poverty of words. I was brought up as a scientist and
– although I take pleasure in poetry and in the lucidity which
scientists can sometimes bring to their work – I feel that words have
in many ways diminished my life.

In the field of philosophy Bacon and Descartes took their discipline away from the contemplation of the uncertainties of living and
sought for a knowledge that could be firmly defined. Schumacher
writes:

While traditional wisdom had considered the human mind as weak but
open-ended, that is capable of reaching beyond itself towards higher and
higher levels, the new thinking took it as axiomatic that the mind's reach
had fixed and narrow limits, which could be clearly determined, while
within those limits it possessed virtually unlimited powers.[1]

Galileo took the matter further. He made clear his belief that
scientific language gives a truer picture of life than ordinary speech:

Philosophy is written in this great book, the universe, which stands continually open to our gaze. But the book cannot be understood unless one first
learns to comprehend the language and read the letters in which it is
composed. It is written in the language of mathematics, and its characters

are triangles, circles, and other geometric figures without which it is humanly impossible to understand a single word of it; without these, one wanders about in a dark labyrinth.[2]

Commenting on this passage, Marjorie Grene writes:

The language of nature, Galileo tells us, is one that we must learn. Certainly; all languages must be learned. But this is a language, he seems to be suggesting, which by no means everybody knows. It is not like one's mother tongue, assimilated in infancy by any normal human child; for certainly he is convinced that at least the wretched Sarsi, against whom his polemic is directed, has never learned it. The language of nature, then, is in some sense a foreign language. And indeed, for most of us, the language of mathematics, which *is* for Galileo nature's language, has to be learned in school, not at home; it is a secondary and artificial acquisition. It belongs, in other words, not to the life world, but to the secondary, painfully constructed world of learning. But how do we learn such a secondary, a foreign language? Either its alphabet is written like our own, and we have to learn the meanings of the words; or there is a foreign alphabet, a different kind of character, to be learned before we can get as far as trying to understand the words. The latter situation holds for nature as Galileo sees it; not even the letters of its language form part of our ordinary environment, but, he insists, we have to learn them too. And again, this is, of course, true of the language of mathematics: we have to familiarize ourselves with its formalisms before we can make use of them in order to understand what they have to teach. To the ordinary person, then, the language of nature bears to the perceptible surface of the things around him a relation rather like that which, for a native English speaker, a page of Chinese or Arabic bears to a page of ordinary English prose. Until he is trained to do so, he cannot make out so much as its constituent elements, let alone their meaning. In short, the universe that 'lies open to our gaze' is, if Galileo is correct, a volume written in a secret code, which only the trained cryptographer can interpret. The rest of us can only 'wander in a dark labyrinth'.[3]

If we transpose these thoughts on to the field of psychotherapy, it is clear that the comparable danger would be to see not triangles and circles but transferences and defences, to reduce the complexity of human interchange to fragmented moves and counter-moves which are then reassembled into an apparently meaningful whole.

The worst ravages upon language in the field of psychology and psychotherapy in recent times have come from the Behaviouristic school of thought. One would expect that those approaches which depend more upon simple, unspecialized appreciation of the other, regarding insight and empathy as important means of understanding, would be less opaque. In general I think they are. But it is only a matter of degree. I will give two examples taken from the leading journals of the Freudian and Jungian schools of thought respectively. I do not want to mislead the reader and I would ask him to take into consideration the facts that, on the one hand, examples of this kind of language are no rarity and very easy to find, but, on the other hand, by taking them out of context I give him little chance of interpreting their meaning. What I have in mind is to call attention to the language:

The same applies to the transformation of the action to its opposite, with the composition of opposition with itself yielding the identity transformation, and so once again we have a two-element subgroup. In the case of the intensifier transformation leading to the elementary mechanism of effectualisation, it is natural to introduce reiteration of the intensifier in such a way that the reiteration of the intensifier transformation leads to ever more intense affectualisation. Thus we do not have a finite number of transformations but rather an infinite one under composition. Also, we do not have a natural inverse transformation, and although we could perhaps define one in terms of the neutralisation transformation on which intellectualisation is based, at the present stage of development of the theory this seems rather artificial. Consequently, the most we will want to say here is that we have a semi-group of transformations that are infinite rather than finite.[4]

A point can come, as Meier states, when the exclusive principles between opposite functions get 'less exclusive' and a synthesis can occur to produce a uniting symbol of healing. But how do 'opposite functions' get less exclusive? Could it be that this occurs via union of the auxiliary (second and third) functions that are not quite so opposed? It is often said that analysis proceeds better if one works at development via them, rather than the inferior function *per se*. In fact, the inferior function cannot be integrated. More accurately stated, it lives us, rather than we it.[5]

The writers of these two extracts would not, I suppose, claim to be original thinkers of the first order, nor have they attracted a following. The case is different with those who are capable of original thought and have the intellectual drive and power to create a school of thought with a language of its own. We have to ask ourselves whether the obscurity of such thinkers is a necessary concomitant to the illumination they give us or whether it derives so much from narcissistic indulgence (or even from a deliberate aim to construct an aura of profundity) that we should not allow ourselves to be led by the nose. But it takes both courage and effort to strip the Emperor of (at least some of) his clothes, and few of us have enough of either quality to make the attempt. Therefore we should be grateful for the recent critiques by Roger Scruton[6] and Richard Wollheim[7] of the hitherto apparently unassailable Lacan (see p. 111).

The language of psychotherapy – if such can be said to exist – is not only in its infancy but is evidently very confused. One reason for this is the fact that the theorist, with objectivity in view, has focused on the mind of the 'object' under scrutiny, namely the patient. Following in the footsteps of psychiatry, he concerns himself with clinical entities and abnormal mental states, to which he has added 'mechanisms of defence'. Let us now look at this language. Even if we leave aside the extremities of obscurity which occasionally face us, we have to consider how we can utilize the valuable insights that have been passed on to us by means of unsuitable language without becoming so blinded by it that we lose sight of the person before us.

If a person is in a confused state of mind we will seek to understand the nature and meaning of this confusion, and in the process of so doing, it is likely that we will make simple distinctions. Some of his communications will ring true for us, some not. When, in our daily living, another person's response to us appears to be false we do not (unless we are psychiatrists or psychotherapists) usually think of his state of mind as 'psychopathological'; more likely we would say he is lying or behaving insincerely, assuming that he has a choice in the matter. If, however, his insincerity is intense, appears to be habituated and beyond his awareness and control, we may, varying according to our familiarity with psychotherapeutic terminology, use such terms as 'pathological liar', 'neurotic', 'hysteric', etc. How useful are these concepts? How dangerous?

In view of our tendency to oversimplification, the risk attached to labelling is a large one. We can all too readily slip from saying, 'He is behaving hysterically', to 'He is a hysteric', or 'He suffers from hysteria', particularly if we are angry with him and seek to justify our anger by discrediting him as a whole. As Szasz[8] has pointed out, the relabelling of certain people as 'hysterics' rather than 'malingerers' has done them more harm than good. It would seem that when a person manifests a characteristic that we do not admire, our tendency is to pin a degrading label on him, thereby corrupting our appreciation of his true being. Bearing in mind the potential destructiveness let us now look at its possible advantages to the thera-

pist. Words such as 'lying', 'scheming', 'insincere', 'superficial', refer
to uncreative ways of behaving, and are helpful, if used accurately,
in understanding people. It would seem, therefore, only a small and
realistic step to construct a vocabulary of terms which might be of
comparable use in describing the behaviour of those who are so
manifestly disturbed and confused that they have engendered a desire
in certain people ('psychotherapists') to elucidate their problems.

Few psychotherapists would, I imagine, seriously challenge the
truth embodied in Freud's concept of 'defence' or 'resistance',
however much they may quibble with the form in which he
presented it. When someone comes to us for help we are reasonably
safe in assuming that whatever else is of import and significance in
our relationship, he will, at times, tend to resist those truths about
himself which he finds distasteful. Because this tendency is so
widespread it would be misleading to call it abnormal. But there is
no doubt – and we are indebted to psychoanalysis for pursuing this
point – that it is a dangerous habit which, if carried to excess, can
lead to disturbingly dissociated (split) states of mind.

The belief that evasion of the truth and lack of wholeness are evils
is central both to contemporary psychotherapeutic theory and to
religious thought, but the former has, I think, clarified the relationship between the two in a new and valuable way. We have, in
the psychoanalytic books and journals of this century, a vast literature on the origins, varieties, and vicissitudes of dissociation and,
provided that it can be done without resort to crippling categoriza-
tion, the continued study of the subject is surely of use. One of the
tasks before us is, wherever possible, to reformulate or replace
these concepts with those which have their basis in ordinary
language and experience.

Although certain forms of dissociation (hysteria, obsessionality,
phobia, etc.) are to an extent arbitrary conceptions, they have a
limited value in that they describe states of mind which occur with
sufficient consistency to enable one person to (sometimes) convey,
in shorthand, an observation which is not *necessarily* misleading. If
I were to say, for example, that Mr X's way of living was obsessional, the reader may get the picture of someone who tended
towards 'conscientiousness, tidiness, meanness, pedantry, rationality, combined with cluelessness about human emotions, respect for
the letter rather than the spirit of the law and for red-tape rather
than creative achievement'[9] and I would have made my point as in

no other way, even if Mr X fell short of all the attributes named in this list. And if I were to say that Mr X suffered from obsessional symptoms, then compulsions such as excessive washing of hands would probably come to mind. If, however, I were to pronounce Mr X to be an 'obsessional neurotic', I would be on more shaky ground, for I may unwittingly convey that I have, by this conception, summed up the whole man or made a diagnosis of established accuracy comparable, say, to that of typhoid fever. It is likely that, in the future, there will be an increase in the number of illnesses (such as cerebral syphilis) known to have organic origins and to reveal a complex of symptoms that would make a medical diagnosis possible. Traditional psychiatry is based upon this assumption. But, whereas this hope justifies continued research into neuropathology, it is clearly dangerous if allowed – as unfortunately is the case – to dominate the psychiatrist's attitude to his patient. The harmful consequences of this approach to disturbed people are horrifying. But it is less – in most countries – the manifestation of a religious or political witch-hunt than the result of naïve overconfidence in 'scientific' theory. The limitation – and, indeed, misleading tendency – of the terms under scrutiny comes from an oversimplified belief in the origins of the state of mind in question: too few ideas are asked to do too much work. In psychiatry and psychoanalysis this tendency has taken different forms, but I am here only concerned with the latter, where the tendency to oversimplify the origins of disability has led to the excessive use of a limited number of 'mechanisms of defence'. We may, as an example, take the notion of 'paranoia'. Paranoia is a term which is now part of our common speech. Indeed, today's paper even proffers a definition. Nicholas de Jongh, the art critic, writes in the *Guardian*: 'Paranoia, in its non-clinical definition, describes a state of mind which fails to distinguish between the possible and the likely.' This is apt; but we could, I think, add to it. Although de Jongh implies that the possibilities in question are unpleasant, hostile ones, he does not actually say so. Moreover, he does not include, in his definition, the characteristic reaction of the person possessed by paranoia: hostility. It would therefore be more accurate to say: 'Paranoia describes a state of mind which fails to distinguish between possible and likely harm, and reacts to the anticipated hazard with hostility.' Thus the person who is in a paranoid frame of mind is *unduly* suspicious and watchful, *unduly* preoccupied with and ready to defend his position or to attack whoever or whatever could be a possible threat. Viewed in this way there is no clear distinction between 'paranoia' and 'non-paranoia', merely a continuum in which we can all find a place. It is a description of experience and behaviour, similar, say, to 'suspiciousness' or 'prickliness' but having a more thorough definition and backed by a more comprehensive, exploratory literature. It gives no indication of the *origin* of the paranoid state of mind. And that is as it should be, for we are concerned with the description of an experience, whatever its origins. By contrast the psychoanalytic definition of 'paranoia' and 'paranoid'[10] focuses on *a single* defensive mechanism, namely projection, which is assumed to account for the experience. The consequences of this error are serious: the patient finds that the subtleties of his anguish remain unseen. It would take us too far from the present discussion to point out the many different origins of the state of mind we call paranoid, but they would appear to include the following.

Firstly, a person's actual or imagined weakness may lead him to view the world as a more dangerous place than it really is. Secondly, a parent may either under- or over-expose the child to the outer world, and, because of the tendency of an overprotective parent to deny anxiety, it is likely that he will fail to shield his child in certain respects; in either event the child will develop an excessive fear of the unfamiliar. Thirdly, someone who has developed a rigid attitude towards certain areas of potentially disruptive experience (e.g. anger) needs to maintain a carefully balanced state of equilibrium; he lives on a knife-edge; his uneasiness derives not only from a fear of specific repressed experience or of anything which reminds him of this experience (as, for instance, when the sight of a corpse might conjure up one's murderous wishes) but of anything which disturbs the even tenor of his life; thus he will fear the unforeseen, though it be apparently harmless and have no malignant symbolic significance. Fourthly, the degree to which a person feels persecuted is related to his basic expectations of life: if he believes that normal experience is free from pain and frustration, then he will be unable to take suffering in his stride but will regard himself as singularly unfortunate – something has occurred which should not (in his view) have occurred, and it must be corrected immediately; he cannot accept the suffering and patiently wait until it is relieved. Consequently he becomes intensely preoccupied with the conditions responsible for the suffering, the possible remedies, develops a sense of grievance that something unnaturally painful has taken place, and manifests symptoms of 'hypochondriasis' or 'paranoia' according to the apparent source of his pain.

I have not chosen to use the term 'paranoia' as an example because it is particularly confused. Indeed, compared to the concept of 'hysteria' it appears rather straightforward. The point I wish to emphasize is that the origins of 'paranoid anxiety' are various and are often not far removed from the kind of thinking that we use in ordinary living when trying to understand and protect ourselves from our fellow-men, and that to focus upon one particular mechanism – 'projection' – is misleading, however ingeniously the idea may be stretched in order to cover the facts. By such means man becomes a psychic skeleton, the equivalent of the matrix of triangles and cubicles through which Galileo saw nature.

Although the rigorous pursuit of precise formulations and definitions of the clinical concepts used in psychotherapy is a worthy undertaking, one wonders if it has merely muddled our understanding of the process; whether it derives more from an unhealthy need for intellectual control of a difficult area of life than a realistic attempt to throw light on the subject. We would, I believe, be much better advised to stay nearer the actual experience. As I write this, I find myself thinking of being with someone whom I might consider to be 'paranoid'. What does this mean in the immediate situation? I imagine him to be in a state of fearful defiance. What does he need? Surely, help in trusting me and an understanding that his defiance may well be a defensive cover for his vulnerability. If he can trust me, if he can show his anguish nakedly, he will no longer be paranoid. It is, I feel, on the basis of a simple descriptive formulation of this kind, put in ordinary language, that elaborations of the concept should be made. This may involve a fresh start. But a fresh start may not be a bad thing; the benefit to be gained from discarding such a misused and dangerous term as 'paranoid' should not be underestimated.

The question is a difficult one. We have to consider whether to improve or abandon the special language of psychopathology. The Freudian school of thought is certainly an advance on the sterility of traditional psychiatry in that it has moved away from conceptions of illness towards conceptions of defensive manoeuvres (attempts to avoid or lessen the impact of a painful reality at the expense of truth). Defence measures are infinite in their variety. Attempts have been made, based on the work of Freud (see, for example, Anna Freud,[11] Fenichel,[12] Nunberg[13]), or, more recently – and focused on the notion of early splitting mechanisms – Fairbairn,[14] and Klein,[15] to order them systematically. But such efforts, although sometimes illuminating, tend, by their reliance on a small number of concepts (e.g. introjection, projection, splitting), to seriously impair the therapist's receptivity to the variety of pretences, ploys, games, and subtleties of expression (e.g. coyness, irony, complacency) which constitute a retreat from the authentic – manoeuvres which are the bread-and-butter of daily life as well as the subject of study by artistic genius.

It is difficult to feel assured that one language is incontestably superior to another, especially in areas that lie outside the physical sciences, and therefore we must be cautious before discarding one. The language of psychopathology, however inadequate, not only has its particular hold on the truth but provides a framework of thought which practitioners can use, should they choose to do so. If, however, we adopt, *in toto*, the theory on which the language is based, rather than using certain important insights encased within it, the sacrifice is great, not least because we will have manufactured an illusion of certainty.

A recent book, Roy Schafer's *A New Language for Psychoanalysis*, brings closer the possibility of using Freud's insights without accepting the whole package. Schafer (who has been markedly influenced by the later Wittgenstein) believes that Freudian theory can be salvaged by a radical operation. His solution is to provide a language which remains close to common speech but possesses a rigorous set of rules for use in the psychoanalytical set-up. He calls this 'action language':

We shall regard each psychological process, event, experience, or behaviour as some kind of activity, henceforth to be called action, and shall designate each action by an active verb stating its nature and by an adverb (or adverbial locution), when applicable, stating the mode of this action.

Adopting this rule entails that, insofar as it is possible to do so sensibly, we shall not use nouns and adjectives to refer to psychological processes, events, etc. In this, we should avoid substantive designations of actions as well as adjectival or traitlike designations of modes of action. Thus, we should not use such phrases as a 'strong ego', 'the dynamic unconscious', 'the inner world', 'libidinal energy', 'rigid defense', 'an intense emotion', 'autonomous ego function', and 'instinctual drive'. This radical departure

from accustomed designations is what it takes really to discontinue physio-
chemical and biological modes of psychological thinking. The essential
referents of these designations will, however, be preserved in other terms.[16]

Two possible (and related) advantages of the new language are
that not only does it render obsolete the inappropriate terminology
of Freud but, in practice, it makes it more difficult for people to
conceal the real meaning of their words behind a veil of apparent
passivity:

People often use substantive metaphors and the passive voice in order to
protect the listener-recipient, and perhaps themselves as well, against
minor and major 'shocks'. For example, to say, 'It's time for me to be
leaving,' might make a leave-taking tolerable or less offensive than simply
to say, 'I'm going now.' Of the various forms of eloquence, some of the
most powerful are mono-syllabic, unadorned, and brief. Less can be
more.[17]

But Schafer recognizes that, at least in ordinary living, indirect-
ness can be of value. He states that:

. . . everyday language is not only a record of the fundamental, unconsciously maintained desires and conflicts with which people are concerned,
but also a record of the many modes that people have developed to ease
subjective distress. I particularly have in mind distress felt in connection
with being held responsible.
   We do use disclaimers to help us 'get off the hook'. With their help we are
able to think and talk about difficult issues in a muted, closed manner. We
use them to protect relationships, to care for the other person as well as
ourselves. For example, when a person says 'understandingly' to a friend
who has disappointed and angered him or her by forgetting an appoint-
ment, 'It must have slipped your mind,' rather than, 'You forgot me,' or,
when one says about one's own forgetting, 'It slipped my mind,' rather
than, 'I forgot you,' one is in either case protecting the relationship. At least
one of the parties is being absolved of responsibility or guilt. To speak
plainly of one's 'forgetting' the other, unless it is a seduction to a gratifying
sado-masochistic interaction, is the sort of directness that ordinarily leads
to a quick deterioration of relationships.[18]

If Schafer's suggestions were carried out, psychoanalysts would
rid themselves of much confusing and irritating jargon, and write in
a way that was closer to common speech; in addition, they would
have a more effective mode of language with which to confront the
extraordinarily persistent efforts of disturbed people to relinquish

their capacity to be. There are, however, certain reservations to make about his idea.

Firstly, his renunciation of nouns and adjectives is radical to an unnecessary degree. This criticism has been well put by Rycroft:

Personally, I feel that Schafer has overstated his case by appearing at times to be trying to eliminate all nouns and adjectives from psychoanalysis. Although it is true that abstract nouns lend themselves to reification and that it is all too easy to persuade oneself that one has explained something by invoking substantive concepts like perverse sexuality, intense aggression, or severe superego when referring to the fact that people act perversely, aggressively, or self-punitively, Schafer seems at times unaware that many nouns are in fact the gerunds and participles of verbs, and that it is only a convention of syntax that transforms them into nouns; the words 'agent' and 'action' being themselves good examples of this process. What he is really rejecting, I think, is the use of nouns that cannot be referred back easily to a verb requiring a person as its subject.[19]

Secondly, he falls between two stools. The changes which he believes necessary are not confined to the language of psychoanalysis but extend to that of ordinary usage. We all deceive ourselves and others by means of verbal manoeuvres which enable us to withhold responsibility for what we are really saying. But Schafer does not make clear the degree to which he believes that the new language of psychoanalysis need depart from an action language suitable to everyday living. The question of 'disclaimed action' is central to this issue. He believes that the plain speaking of action language in the psychoanalytic setting involves 'the sort of directness that ordinarily leads to a quick deterioration of relationships'. But we have to ask ourselves whether the messy language that helps preserve our relationships in ordinary life may *also* have a place in psychotherapy.

Thirdly, Schafer's radicalism does not extend to a criticism of the belief that a (Freudian) formal, scientific, logical, systematic, and finely ordered framework is sufficient to encompass the therapeutic encounter. He leaves us (despite his own disclaimers) with the impression of an austerity that is rather forbidding, a purism that appears liable to omit the flesh and blood of human intercourse and a tendency to be directive – to structure the setting in a way which may *encourage* the passivity he so wishes to eliminate. The reader will have to go to Schafer himself (a journey well worth taking) to decide whether this impression is correct, but I will give one example. Referring to the question of the language in which the analyst's communication to his patient should be forged Schafer suggests that in place of, 'Say everything that comes to mind', the analyst should 'Convey the sense of the following ideas':

I shall expect you to talk to me each time you come. As you talk, you will notice that you refrain from saying certain things. You may do so because you want to avoid being trivial, irrelevant, embarrassed, tactless, or otherwise disruptive. It is essential to our work that you do this as little as possible. I urge you to tell me of those instances of selection or omission no matter what their content may be.[20]

The difference in formulation does not seem of great moment. We are left with the more important question: 'Should the therapist so structure the relationship that the patient feels an obligation to talk or behave in a certain way?' There is a sense in which Schafer may actually increase the patient's obligation to do so. In his critique of action language Meissner writes:

One fundamental issue embedded in this question of the nature of theory is the attitude taken towards experience. The attitude of the action-language approach is to see the patient's account as if it were the text to be interpreted. The patient reports something, but the question is not *what* does he report, but *why* does he report it and report it in that way. The patient's experience is thus accepted as a report rather than as a fact. If the patient reports a certain passivity or suffering in his emotional experience, the action-language approach makes a presumption of activity and responsibility and wants to know the reasons why the patient would give such a passive and victimized account.[21]

Thus action language, by focusing the therapist's attention so sharply on the interpretation of verbal behaviour, may heighten the barrier between himself and his patient. Therefore, despite his originality and rigour, Schafer has not freed the analyst from the grip of a scientific conception of man.

Paulo Freire has written of the 'invasiveness' of a language which is not endogenous to the society, and we should, I think, be similarly aware of the invasiveness of a specialized psychotherapeutic language. The nearer we stay to common speech the less likely we are to destroy the meaning of those who seek our help. Personally I would not take this dictum to the extent of a veto. The psychotherapeutic set-up is an unusual one and experiences occur within it which sometimes highlight features which pass unnoticed in ordin-

ary life. When we speak to clients we do not always need a special
term to describe these features, but if we are to generalize from our
experience, then some words may be added to our daily vocabulary.
However, these words (or phrases) may be *very few* in number.
Obvious examples are 'transference', 'countertransference', and
'therapeutic regression'.

Even with these few concepts we must be cautious, for much of
the experience that they connote can be expressed in simple words.
For instance, long before the term 'therapeutic regression' was
coined, William James wrote of a state that:

by getting so exhausted with the struggle that we have to stop, – so we drop
down, give up, and *don't care* any longer. Our emotional brain-centres
strike work, and we lapse into a temporary apathy. Now there is
documentary proof that this state of temporary exhaustion not infrequently
forms part of the confession crisis. So long as the egoistic worry of the sick
soul guards the door, the expansive confidence of the soul of faith gains no
presence. But let the former faint away, even for a moment, and the latter
can profit by the opportunity, and, having once acquired possession, may
retain it.[22]

In seeking for an ordinary way of describing psychotherapy we
are faced, time and again, with the problem of finding our way
between the 'hard', obsessionally neat formulations of the scientist
and the 'soft', flowery words of those who write about their work
with naïve sentimentality. The task is comparable to that of writing
good poetry. The man-in-the-street may be moved by a sunset as
deeply as the poet but if he tries to describe his emotions he will
likely utter banalities. The psychotherapist who attempts to convey
the significant experiences in his work will almost certainly lack the
necessary poetic gift, yet he can no more improve his communication by resorting to special language than can the poet. He can only
write as clearly and truthfully as possible, recognizing that to take
cover behind the aridity of the conventional, objective 'case-
history' may ensure professional respectability but lead him into the
fatal error described by Blake:

> He who bends to himself a joy
> Doth the winged life destroy:

But there is a further difficulty. Although we might decide to rely
for the most part on ordinary words, our total communication (the

gestalt of our expression) can still be distorted by special techniques which inhibit communication. The priest may give up his Latin but retain his priestly voice, the parallel of which is the psychotherapist's measured, unemotional tone. And those of us who aim to escape from this position may easily find ourselves straining towards an opposite one that is equally inauthentic. The clergyman in the pub who feels obliged to convey, 'Look, I'm not really a Holy Man. See me drinking my pint of bitter', has his unfortunate counterpart in the psychotherapist who says, 'I'm not a stuck-up Freudian. I'm Joe. Let's get together.' But, although there are few limits to our ability to elude the authentic and creative, I believe we have more hope of doing so if we recognize the need to divest ourselves as far as possible of a professional language – whether verbal or non-verbal – which cloaks our true being.

Note

Jacques Lacan is a rather special case. His fragmentation of ordinary discourse is motivated by the structuralist aim of undermining the concept of autonomous self. Whether or not we agree with his view we may still find his means to an end unacceptably destructive and suspect that he is a victim of his own delight in word-play.

References

1. Schumacher, E. F. (1977), *A Guide for the Perplexed*, Jonathan Cape, London.
2. Grene, Marjorie (1965), *Approaches to a Philosophical Biology*, Basic Books, New York, p. 10.
3. Ibid., p. 11.
4. Suppes, P. and Warren, H. (1975), 'On the Generation and Classification of Defence Mechanisms', *Int. J. Psycho-anal.* 56. 405.
5. Edinger, E. F. (1960), 'The Ego-self Paradox', *J. Anal. Psychology*, 5. 3.
6. Scruton, R. (1978), 'Incantations of the Self', *Times Literary Supplement*, 11 August.
7. Wollheim, R. (1979), *New York Review of Books*.
8. Szasz, T. (1961), *The Myth of Mental Illness*, Harper & Row, New York.
9. Rycroft, C. (1968), *A Critical Dictionary of Psychoanalysis*, Nelson, London.
10. Ibid.

11. Freud, A. (1937), *The Ego and the Mechanisms of Defence*, Hogarth, London.
12. Fenichel, O. (1946), *The Psychoanalytical Theory of Neurosis*, Routledge and Kegan Paul, London.
13. Nunberg, H. (1955), *The Principles of Psychoanalysis*, International Universities Press, New York.
14. Fairbairn, W. R. D. (1952), *Psychoanalytic Studies of the Personality*, Tavistock, London.
15. Klein, M. (1948), *Contributions to Psychoanalysis*, Hogarth, London.
16. Schafer, R. (1976), *A New Language for Psychoanalysis*, Yale University Press, New Haven.
17. Ibid.
18. Ibid.
19. Rycroft, C. (1976), *New York Review of Books*, 27 May.
20. Schafer, R., *A New Language for Psychoanalysis*.
21. Meissner, W. W. (1979), 'Methodological Critique of Action Language', *J. American Psychoanalytical Assoc.*
22. James, W. (1904), *The Varieties of Religious Experience*, Longmans, Green & Co., London.

8. Uncertainty

Shortly after dawn, or what would have been dawn in a
normal sky, Mr. Artur Sammler with his bushy eye took in
the books and papers of his West Side bedroom and
suspected strongly that they were the wrong books, the
wrong papers. In a way it did not matter much to a man of
seventy-plus, and at leisure. You had to be a crank to insist
on being right. Being right was largely a matter of
explanations. Intellectual man had become an explaining
creature. – Saul Bellow, *Mr. Sammler's Planet*

Although, in keeping with the dominant Western ideal, the
psychotherapist strives for certainty in both his theory and practice,
there exists, as I have already indicated, a powerful tradition in
philosophy which points in the other direction. It is a tradition
which still flourishes, as witnessed by the recent publication of two
lucid and illuminating works: Barrett[1] brings together the relevant
ideas of Kierkegaard, Heidegger, and William James; and Isaiah
Berlin[2] traces the early dissenting voices of Vico, Herder, and
others who pursue the notion of plurality. These trends in philosophy give heart to those of us who, in whatever discipline, find
ourselves outside the prevailing belief in the encompassing truth.

In this chapter I shall continue to explore the possibilities of a
psychotherapeutic approach in which the search for an explanation
is not dominant and confidence in a unified theory is wanting, and
shall begin by asking the question, 'To what extent and in what way
should the therapist convey to his patient a certainty that he knows
what has to be done?' As so often when thinking about psychotherapy a comparison with childhood may be helpful.

The importance to a child of a measure of clarity and consistency
in its parents has been well brought out in the writings of Lidz,
Bateson, Wynne, and others who have studied the families of
'schizophrenic' offspring. Searles, who, with a psychotherapeutic
intensity that possibly surpasses anyone else's, has explored the
problems of schizophrenic patients, is well aware of their need for
an unambiguous environment. He makes the following pertinent
observation:

The child cannot build up realistic perceptions except in so far as there is a
reliable, mutually trusting emotional climate in which he knows where he
stands with each of his parents – knows who he is to them, and knows that

he is loved and accepted by them. In these ['schizophrenogenic] familes there is so little of trustful, leisurely sharing of one another's thinking as to leave little time and emotional security for the weighing of perceptions before meanings must be imposed upon them. Instead a perception has barely been made before it must be reacted to, by both parent and child, as confirming one or another emotional prejudice, one or another rigid superego stan-ard, derived from parental indoctrination. The child is led to feel that not to *know* – to exist in a state of uncertainty and of searching for a meaning – means to be crazy, to be something beyond the human pale.[3]

We are presented with what at first sight appears to be a paradox. The child needs reliability; he needs to know where he stands with his parents; yet at the same time he needs to be allowed 'to exist in a state of uncertainty'. The paradox is resolved if we recognize that the child must be sure that the parents know him (in a basic, over-all way), yet can tolerate the degree to which, being a person and not a mechanism, they can never know him with exactitude. This uncertainty will be reflected in their attitude to life: they know that it is a mystery and they can therefore tolerate ambiguity, irony, and humour. A similar point (including criticism of Bateson's widely known 'double bind' concept and Russell's theory of types on which the concept is based) has been made by Kafka.[4]

The consequences of an inability to tolerate uncertainty are not confined to schizophrenogenic families. Arnold Green, in a paper which has now become a classic, 'The Middle-Class Male Child and Neurosis', describes the traumatic effects of an ever-present watchfulness over children: the family, either by an overt protec-tiveness or by an unspoken assumption about the nature of the child, cripple his ability to act spontaneously.

Green writes:

Modern 'scientific child care' enforces a constant supervision and diffused worrying over the child's health, eating spinach, and ego-development; this is complicated by the fact that much energy is spent forcing early walking, toilet-training, talking, because in an intensively competitive milieu middle-class parents from the day of birth on are constantly comparing their own child's development with that of the neighbour's children. The child must also be constantly guarded from the danger of contacting various electrical gadgets and from kicking valuable furniture. The middle-class child's discovery that the living room furniture is more important to his mother than his impulse to crawl over it, unquestionably finds a place in the background of the etiology of a certain type of neurosis, however absurd it may appear.[5]

Green wrote this in 1946 and it is already easy to disassociate ourselves from the kind of upbringing that he describes, but in our increasingly 'abstract' society (to use Zijderveld's term[6]) we continue to find other ways of absorbing our children's spontaneity by a too quick and watchful response.

The zenith of watchfulness is reached in psychotherapy. We listen with great care to the exact words spoken, we observe the gestures, we take notes, we record and videotape our sessions, and we feel the constant pressure to make interpretations and to encapsulate the experience into a theoretical framework. But at what cost? In our quest for certainty are we not in danger of a diminished reverence for the person comparable to the contemporary destruction of the aura of objects of art described by Walter Benjamin?

In speaking of reverence for the other person I do not wish to imply solemnity. In fact, quite the reverse, for reverence and fun often go together; both contain an element of magic and both can be destroyed by the scientific attitude. I would like to give two examples of the problems faced by students of psychotherapy who find themselves puzzled by the phenomenon of play.

Dr A came one day having, the previous evening, seen an opera by which he had been very moved. He tried to describe the feelings it evoked, but in a short while he exclaimed, 'It's impossible! One can't get these things into words.' He was reminded by this of a session with a child the day previously. 'We just played, that's all. It was very good. But I couldn't write it up. There's nothing to write.' I asked him if he believed it has been 'therapeutic' for the child. 'Oh, yes', he said without hesitation; 'That's all I'm sure about.'

Dr B was seeing a woman patient for the first time. She came into the room, looked at the chair provided and said, 'Is this the hot seat?'

'Yes,' he replied. And they both laughed.

However, when the student reported the session to his supervisor the latter exclaimed: 'You should never have said that! That was colluding with the patient's defences.'

There are many arguments to support the supervisor's stance, but I believe him to have been profoundly wrong. The patient was probably well aware of the ironies of the situation, and the cost of a laboured interpretation might have been great.

There is, as I suggested earlier, something very paradoxical about Freud's attitude to science. He had a great respect for art, an awareness of the mystery of existence, and an interest in the un-canny, yet his aim was to bring phenomena to order, to make known what was unknown. In his terms, 'Where id was, there shall ego be.' The beginning of his search for a method has been well described in Ernest Jones's biography.[7] Jones emphasizes two very different influences: firstly, Freud's treatment, described in *Studies in Hysteria*, of the patient Fräulein Elizabeth von R., and secondly the writings of Ludwig Börne.

Fräulein Elizabeth did not respond to hypnotism and Freud pressed her forehead with his hand and asked her to try to recall any memories related to her symptoms. After several attempts the patient did bring out what was in her mind, but with the comment 'I could have told you that the first time, but I didn't think it was what you wanted'. This comment induced Freud to give the strict injunc-ture to ignore all censorship and to express every thought even if she considered it irrelevant, unimportant, or too unpleasant. On one occasion (perhaps a momentous one in the history of psychoanaly-sis) Fräulein Elizabeth reproved Freud for interrupting the flow of her thought by his questions and demanded that he listen – which he then did. Jones describes Freud's step as 'a curious one to have taken: it meant displacing a systematic and purposeful search with a known aim in view by an apparently blind and uncontrolled meandering'.

Jones believes that another important, though undeclared, source of Freud's confidence in the method of free-association was the writings of one of his favourite authors, Ludwig Börne, who had written a book entitled *The Art of Becoming an Original Writer in Three Days*. Börne advises that the prospective writer set down 'without any falsification or hypocrisy, everything that comes into your head'. One of his aphorisms was 'The true act of self-education lies in making oneself unwitting'.

In the method of free-association, described by Freud as the 'fundamental rule' of psychoanalysis, the source of inspiration is changed from doctor to patient. The patient speaks in the manner of a creative artist and the doctor listens, with an open mind, ready to be taught.

Although Freud thereby created a therapeutic model (named by one of his early patients the 'talking treatment') which, in extending the confessional from the priest to the doctor, has had a momentous effect on twentieth-century psychiatry, the exact nature of the listening process that he introduced is not immediately clear. There is no doubt that he had powers of concentration that far surpassed most of his fellow-men, and was able to make extremely penetrating formulations about the nature of the psyche on the basis of his observations of patients. But we are left with the question 'To what extent was his mind really open to the patients?' Or, to put it in terms used earlier in this book, 'Was his attitude one of receptivity to those who sought his help or did he intrude with ideas which derived less from his experience with people (in or out of the consulting room) than his knowledge of current thinking in neurology and biology?' Frank Sulloway, in his carefully researched *Freud, Biologist of the Mind*, suggests that Freud unconsciously attempted to conceal the degree to which his theory was inspired by biology in order to give the impression that it was the unadulterated findings of the psychoanalytic technique, *bona fide* products of empirical science. Quoting from *Studies in Hysteria* Holloway[8] gives evidence of Freud's remorseless pursuit of the supposed sexual origin of his patients' neuroses in the face of their protestations. Although Holloway overstates his case (e.g. he has nothing to say on the origins of Freud's theory of transference) he lends support to the idea that Freud has left us with insights of immense importance about the human mind (however he tumbled upon them) and a model of listening which is not entirely suited to those of us who do not subscribe to the theory of psychic determinism. We who have succeeded Freud have tended to accept his formulations (or those of his early powerful colleagues) of the psyche and we try to understand our patients in terms of the formulations. We, also, have succumbed to the increasing pressure of science, resulting sometimes in a method (such as that described by Viderman, discussed earlier in this book) which even surpasses, in rigour and restriction, Freud's own way of relating to patients.

It is not my purpose to assess Freud's contribution to our understanding of life but rather to make an attempt to determine the adequacy of the current model of psychotherapy which owes so much to his influence. It is, I believe, vital that we do not let ourselves be so impressed by his insights that (a) we assume them to have derived directly from his method and/or (b) we believe that a method which produces such valuable insights is necessarily desirable when it comes to healing. This question is crucial to any discussion about the nature of the therapist's authority. If the therapist is in possession of a specialized knowledge allowing him to perceive his patients with certainty, or if he has a technique for extracting relevant knowledge with certainty, then he may be justified in hiding behind a mask of omnipotence and clarity. If, however, this is not the case, then his authority, like that of his patient, will depend on the quality, in ordinary terms, of his judgement. But we can take heart from the fact that if it is also the case that mankind (whether child or adult) has a natural tolerance of the mystery and ambiguity of experience – a tolerance which has been eroded by contemporary efforts to control nature beyond the bounds of possibility – then the patient will be able to survive the uncertainty of the psychotherapy to a greater degree than is usually recognized. One of the ambiguities he must face is that he has to trust a person who is fallible. He can, I believe, accept this fallibility if he sees that the therapist, no matter what his limitations and peculiarities, has an over-all confidence in and commitment to the therapeutic process and can be relied upon to listen with sound judgement. Let me give an example.

Margaret came to me having had two previous analyses, and began by telling me the circumstances in which she had stopped the second of these. One night she awoke to the sound of rain, and the thought came to her mind: 'This will water Dr X's garden and his plants will grow.' It was surprising, and very pleasing to her, to have, for the first time, a positive warm feeling towards her analyst. During the next session with Dr X she related this thought. 'But he was not at all moved by it,' she said to me sadly. 'He did not seem to realize how important it was that he be able to accept a warm feeling from me.'

For the first two months Margaret behaved in a very regressed way during sessions. Much of the time she curled up on the couch, sometimes in apparent anguish, sometimes crying like a baby or speaking like a very small child. I felt rather unsure of the way to respond to her but at certain times I reacted to her in a manner that was more like a parent to a tiny child than as one adult to another. The result of this was that, in her words, she 'was beginning to come alive'.

Then I went on holiday for three days. Unfortunately, on the journey, an approaching vehicle ran out of control and in the ensuing crash I was injured and taken to hospital. For two months I was unable to work. I wrote to Margaret from hospital suggesting the name of a colleague whom she could see while I was away.

On my return to work I received the full force of Margaret's fury and rejection. 'You should have known there could be no substitute,' she said. 'If only you had thrown out a life-line to me. I needed so little. Just an occasional note so that I knew you were all right and felt in contact. I nearly sent stamped and addressed envelopes and asked you to say, "I'm O.K. Peter". That's all I needed to stop worrying and to be able to hold you in my mind. Now it's gone. I don't know how to get it back.'

I myself was torn between responsive anger to the intensity of her attacks and sympathy with her plight. I think her anger was not entirely unjustified and, given the time again (the time that we always ask for and rarely get), I believe I would act differently. However, after a few weeks we found our presence in the same room to be intolerable and agreed to part company.

Six months later Margaret wrote asking me if we could resume therapy. Her letter cost me a very restless night but I said I would see her, and following the interview – and with the greatest reluctance – agreed to have another go. Margaret, knowing the distress she had managed to cause me ('I seem to know how to hurt people,' she once said) and the emotional risk I felt I was taking in resuming therapy, was very grateful for my decision – and remained so throughout the subsequent therapy. She found it reassuring that such an apparently catastrophic rift could be bridged.

Our second attempt at therapy was at first tentative, laboured, and difficult, and involved an extensive reconstruction of what had happened between us during and after my accident; but gradually mutual trust was re-established. On my side this was now on a more secure basis. I had come to know Margaret much better, to feel safe with her, to respect her determined pursuit of the truth, to appreciate her interest in my own welfare, and to understand that she only became savage when her anguish was intolerable. Also, during the therapy, Margaret came to know me very well. I had not hidden my emotional reactions to her and she learned a lot about my strengths and weaknesses. As we explored her childhood and infantile life and its re-emergence in therapy she realized that much of my understanding of her conflicts came from the experience of my own problems and I told her about my childhood and the ways in which I had succeeded or failed to overcome my difficulties. I feel unable to describe adequately the tenor of our discourse without a lengthy and very detailed account, but I would like to emphasize that these interchanges were made with little reserve. What I gave her was of a much more intimate nature than a purely factual account. And, as she grew to know me better, Margaret developed an increasing urge to help me with my own problems, and did whatever she could, directly or indirectly, to this end. The knowledge that she sometimes succeeded – if only in a minor way – gave her enormous pleasure. There are two points I wish to make in regard to this account.

Firstly, Margaret was not disturbed by the revelations of my failings; she was only disturbed by my failing *her* in a major way. In other words, what was crucial to her was her own judgement, based on her direct experience of me, of my capacity to respond with love, integrity, and understanding to *her*. Given this she could accept the marked degree in which I fell short of omnipotence. Indeed, she gained a feeling of security from the belief that my preparedness to admit my failings increased the possibility of overcoming difficulties between us.

Secondly, the acknowledgement of need on my part reduced her feeling of impotence (derived from early life) in regard to her urge to heal others and made it possible for her sometimes to respond to my needs helpfully. The importance of Margaret's therapeutic striving towards me is, I believe, not an isolated, unusual, phenomenon. The traditional assumption that the analyst is well and the patient ill and that the therapeutic process is a one-way flow has for too long obscured from view the patient's urge to help the therapist. But in a recent paper, with the illumination characteristic of his writings, Searles has unearthed this urge. He suggests that:

. . . the patient *is ill because, and to the degree that*, his own psychotherapeutic strivings have been subjected to such vicissitudes that they have been rendered inordinately intense, frustrated of fulfillment or even acknowledgement, admixed therefore with unduly intense components of hate, envy and competitiveness; and subjected, therefore, to repression. In transference terms, the patient's illness expresses his unconscious attempt to cure the doctor.[9]

I would like to remind the reader that Margaret came to me because, in her view, her analyst failed to acknowledge or respond to her sudden, unexpected thought, 'The rain will fall on his garden and make his plants grow.' I would suggest (from the advantage point to which a subsequent therapist is always privileged) that Margaret was expressing not only warm feelings towards her analyst but therapeutic strivings. And I would further suggest that not only is it of vital importance (as Searles believes) to acknowledge such strivings but that it can be appropriate to allow the patient the fullest opportunity to learn the ways in which he may help the therapist – and to respond to such help. This can only occur if the therapist reveals his true nature, as far as is within his power to do so.

I will end this description by allowing Margaret to speak for herself. I sent the above account to her asking if it was accurate. She replied that (except for one minor detail, which I have amended) it was, and her letter contained the following observations. Having commented on the usefulness, in her view, of my openness to her, which contrasted sharply with her own background ('When nothing was brought out into the open and freely talked about'), she writes:

Two examples come to mind. One day I picked up a feeling of sadness and you told me that your sister had died very suddenly. You said you were glad I was there that afternoon. I had picked up the feeling of sadness and for once just being there and being me had helped in a small way. Another time I asked you how you were and you said that you had just discovered that your bank balance was lower than expected. Not something any of us like but no major disaster and certainly nothing to do with me because I had paid my bill! We just had a laugh about it and it gave me a sense of proportion. This kind of thing happened many times but it was the fact that you told me the truth that helped. If you had brushed my questions aside I should have wasted a lot of time speculating and wasting the session. In the event such interchanges always lead to closer contact. After a while I didn't need to ask all the time if you were all right.

Incidentally, I remember very vividly two occasions when I picked up a special feeling of happiness. These were a great gift because such occurrences were rare in my childhood.

It had never disturbed me to know that you still have problems that need working on. It works the opposite way. It means so much to know that you understand these deep areas from your own experience and that you have learned to cope with them. That you can allow yourself to be vulnerable and in need of support so that you know how to give support in a real way to your patients. It has always encouraged me and given me confidence to know that you are still growing.

One way of formulating the problem of those who seek help is to say that, because of an illusory belief in certainty, they have difficulty in maintaining reasonable control of their lives. They either (obsessionally) attempt an excessively tight and limited organization or (hysterically) are impulsive and unrestrained to a degree that is harmful – and often alternate between these two extremes. If the patient is to be helped the therapy must not itself suffer from the same symptom.

The Encounter Movement would seem to derive from a healthy attempt to escape from the undue control not only of traditional Freudian analysis but of the cultural mores of the nineteenth and early twentieth centuries. Unhappily, in this endeavour, it has (it seems to me) fallen prey to the opposite danger: it plays into the hands of those of us who seek to escape reality by denying the fact that humility is essential to the gradual and very complex journey to our understanding of each other.

The insensitivity of a precipitate, arrogant, and inappropriate confrontation is beautifully described in a scene in Turgenev's *Rudin*. Rudin and Natalya have just discovered that they are in love with each other. But both are aware that Volyntsev has nourished hopes, for a long time, of gaining Natalya's heart. Rudin, who believes earnestly in being sincere with people, decides to speak of the matter to Volyntsev:

'I came to you as one honourable man to another,' repeated Rudin, 'and I now want to submit my case to your judgement . . . I trust you completely . . .'

'What is it all about, then?' asked Volyntsev, who remained standing in his former position and glared morosely at Rudin, occasionally pulling the ends of his moustache.

'Permit me to explain . . . I came in order to clear things up, naturally; but that can't be done all at once.'

'Why not?'

'A third person is involved . . .'

'What third person?'

'Sergey Pavlych, you know what I mean.'

'Dmitry Nikolaich, I haven't the slightest idea what you mean.'

'As you wish . . .'

'I wish you'd speak plainly!' Volyntsev broke in.

He was beginning to lose his temper in real earnest.

Rudin frowned.

'Very well . . . we're alone . . . I must tell you – besides, you've no doubt already guessed' (Volyntsev impatiently shrugged his shoulders) '. . . I must tell you that I love Natalya Alexeyevna and have the right to suppose that she also loves me.'

Volyntsev went pale, but instead of answering walked over to the window and stood with his back to the room.

'You understand, Sergey Pavlych,' Rudin went on, 'that if I weren't sure . . .'

'Of course!' Volyntsev briskly interrupted, 'I don't doubt in the least . . . Splendid! Here's to you! I'm just staggered at what the devil made you think of coming to me with this news of yours . . . What's it got to do with me? Why should it concern me whom you love or who loves you? I simply can't understand it.'

Volyntsev continued to stare out of the window. His voice sounded hollow.

Rudin stood up.

'I will tell you, Sergey Pavlych, why I decided to come to you and why I didn't consider I even had the right to hide from you . . . our mutual disposition. I have too deep a respect for you – that's why I came; I didn't want . . . neither of us wanted to act out a comedy in front of you. Your feeling for Natalya Alexeyevna was known to me . . . Believe me, I know what I'm worth; I know how unworthy I am to take your place in her heart; but if this has been destined to happen, would it have been better to cheat and deceive and pretend? Would it have been better to submit to misunder-standings or even the possibility of a scene like the one at dinner yesterday? Sergey Pavlych, tell me.'

Volyntsev folded his arms in front of him as if forcibly holding back his feelings.

'Sergey Pavlych!' Rudin continued, 'I feel I've annoyed you . . . but try and understand us . . . try and understand we didn't have any other way of showing you our respect, of showing you that we know how to appreciate your directness and nobility of soul. Frankness, complete frankness would have been inappropriate with someone else, but with you it be-comes an obligation. It's nice for us to think that our secret is in your hands . . .'

Volyntsev broke into forced laughter.

'Thanks for entrusting me with it!' he exclaimed, 'although, I ask you to take note, I wanted neither to know your secret nor to entrust you with mine, but you're treating it anyhow as your own property.'

Soon after Rudin's departure Volyntsev is visited by his friend Lezhnev and tells him what has just occurred.

'Well, my dear chap, you've astonished me,' declared Lezhnev as soon as Volyntsev had finished. 'I'd come to expect a good many eccentricities from him, but this . . . Still, I can recognise him even in this.'

'You don't say!' said an excited Volyntsev. 'It's a bloody liberty! I almost threw him through the window! Did he want to come and show off in front of me, or did he get cold feet? What was it all for? How can one make up one's mind to go and see someone . . .'

Volyntsev put his hands behind his head and fell silent.

'No, my dear chap, it's not that,' Lezhnev retorted calmly. 'You won't believe me, but he did it with the best of intentions. Really and truly . . . it was to be both noble and candid, can't you see? and, well, there was an opportunity for talking, of giving vent to a little eloquence; and that's what his type need, they can't live without it . . .'

Although Rudin comes out badly in this episode, Turgenev clearly has much sympathy for his inept idealism, a sympathy which appears later in the book. But it is Rudin's arrogant sense of *certainty* and his narcissistic preoccupation with his own performance which let him down. A century and a half later we are still faced, in circumstances which are very different from those familiar to Turgenev, with similar problems in our current attempts to formulate a method of approaching those who are disturbed.

In everday life we do not always confront each other with the naked truth. Thinkers of a cynical bent (in fields of philosophy, psychology, psychotherapy, and literature) have made much of this fact and constructed theories of human interaction upon it. But the motives for concealment are not *always* unworthy and are often very realistic.

We know (for we have been told by people wiser than ourselves) that the way to truth is a long, difficult, and wild one: there are no short cuts, no tricks available, and no profit to be gained from an attempt to convert it to the regularities of a municipal footpath. In other words, we do best to rely, in deciding how much to reveal of ourselves, on our day-to-day judgement rather than an ideology, for ideology can blind us to the actual needs of the other, and our own capacity (or lack of it) to answer them.

There is a significant difference between a theory, ideology, or ritual based on the belief that one person (or a group of people) knows what is best for another, and the acceptance, by the two parties, of conventions which are negotiable and do not mystify.

Every meeting between two people involves both possibility and limitation. What can occur is restricted not only by individual caution and inhibition but by social structures and conventions and the tendency of people to transform some of their spontaneous actions into mutually acceptable moves. One very obvious limiting factor is verbal communication: however gifted we may be with words and however sensitive to intonations, we have to stay close to the path that has already been mapped out for us. Structures of this kind are necessary because human beings do not possess the equipment to restructure their social perceptions continually, and even if they had this capacity it would absorb a colossal amount of energy and make their lives even more uncertain than they are at present. The conflict between control and freedom, discipline and permissiveness, regulation and autonomy is an age-old conflict and one despairs of finding any satisfactory solution; yet everywhere we turn we are faced with the problem afresh.

The simplification involved in a psychotherapeutic convention ensures that too much energy is not wasted on inessentials and, in addition, it brings the sense of security which accompanies ritual. To the extent that formalization occurs the psychotherapist has a function comparable to that of a priest taking part in a religious ceremony: he acts not as himself but as an agent whose personal life and preoccupations can, for the moment, be forgotten; by this means he not only preserves himself from a scrutiny which might detract from his performance but enables all concerned to focus on matters which are difficult to approach in the muddle and turmoil of ordinary living. We need, however, to continually question the degree to which, in any particular encounter, formality is justified or not. Let me give two examples of the kind of dilemma which the therapist may face in this connection.

A young man asked me whether, during his next session, I will allow him to use my piano and listen to his play. This departure from our present formal arrangement may bring problems. My consulting room has been built on as a unit which is separate from the house itself. So in order that he may play the piano I would have to invite him into the 'private' part of the house where he might meet other members of my family, a move which may be seen by him as the beginnings of a different kind of relationship – a social rather than professional one. On the other hand, I felt inclined to agree to his suggestion because he may have a need to express something to me which he could not do with words in the room – but in permitting this innovation I take a risk that the change in the boundary between us could cause confusion, be used by him to make it more difficult for me to say the kind of hard things from which an ordinary friend may shrink, and increase the possibility that the final ending of our relationship may be felt less as a normal professional move than a personal rejection. And I take the further risk in that I may hate his piano-playing and be unable to conceal my distaste.

The second example is taken from the early stages of therapy with a man who does not know what moves to make in order to contact people and is terrified of alienating them by a gesture that would be unacceptable.

After his second or third session I went for my weekly swim at the public pool nearby, and we met each other in the changing room. After the next session he said, 'Are you swimming this afternoon?' I answered, 'Yes, I had thought of doing so.' 'Shall we go together?' he asked; 'My car is outside and I can take you'.

For several reasons my impulse was to say 'No'. Firstly, my swim is a relaxed time when I can forget about psychotherapy. Secondly, because I adhere to the policy of keeping professional and social relationships apart when possible, I foresaw an unwelcome complication to the therapy. However, if I declined to join him I might inflict on him a hurtful wound at an early stage of our relationship.

At every turn, as in ordinary living, the therapist has to make complex decisions of this kind. Should he expose his being to the patient or protect him from knowledge of his imperfections and incompatible views? Should he openly (and, at least truthfully) state that he intends to hide himself?

We have already found this dilemma in the discussion of transference (Chapter 4) in which I suggested that the concept, however illuminating, can readily be invoked to protect the therapist: in presenting himself as a screen for the projections of the patient, he can hide his vulnerabilities without recognizing the true motives of his stance. It is not too difficult to pinpoint this fallacy. More of a problem is the question – on which I have focused in this chapter – of the degree to which patients need to be protected from the recognition of their therapist's vulnerabilities because they simply could not deal with them. I have suggested that, in this matter, we are in danger of overprotecting our patients, not only out of a need to preserve our own self-esteem but from a misguided philosophy of living. It must be noted, however, that this suggestion runs counter to an important trend in current thinking.

The Freudian belief – creatively extended by Winnicott – that it is therapeutically necessary for certain patients to pass through a period in which they are supported by their trust in an idealized therapist is likely to influence us in the direction of reticence and concealment. If, as a child, someone has missed an essential experience of security due to 'environmental failure' then he will need to relive it in the therapeutic encounter: he will regress from a position of pseudo-independence and come to rely, for a period of time, on someone who will act as a substitute parent. To the extent that he needs 'holding' the therapist must not intrude with his own feelings and problems. Winnicott[10] is very clear on this point and sets before us a model of patience and restraint that many will find hard to follow. I am sure that there are many occasions when such a course is correct. But I believe that it should not be set up as a paradigm for, as such, it involves the debatable theory that an infant lives in a state of illusion. In fact, our knowledge of the way a baby experiences life has no secure foundation. Our memories, reconstructions, and observations still leave open wide gaps which we fill with guesswork. According to the accepted view the infant fails to recognize the fact that he and his mother are separate objects. And the word 'illusion' is used to describe (see, for example, Marian Milner's admirable account of the analysis of a 'schizophrenic' patient, *The Hands of the Living God*[11]) the state of mind – common to infancy, creativity, mental illness, and regressive states in analysis – in which the more ordinary vision of the world is replaced by a sense of fusion between self and other. I find this theory misleading, and would suggest that the person in such a state of mind has an awareness of a psychological union which actually exists, and is making a selection from experiences just as valid as that which enables us logically to separate the things around us. In other words, the child – and the regressed patient in therapy – has a more realistic grasp of the *essential* nature of a relationship than we give him credit for. Our response should be less a matter of protecting him from the relationship – although at times we may do this – than offering him, if we have it to offer, the reality of our ordinary warmth and understanding.

References

1. Barrett, W. (1979), *The Illusion of Technique*, William Kimber, London.
2. Berlin, I. (1979), *Against the Current*, Hogarth, London.

3. Searles, H. (1979), *Countertransference and Related Subjects*, International Universities Press, New York.
4. Kafka, U. S. (1972), 'Paradox, Time and Object Constancy', paper read to the British Psychoanalytical Society, 15 March 1972.
5. Green, A. W. (1960), 'The Middle-Class Male Child and Neurosis', in *A Modern Introduction to the Family*, ed. Bell, N. W. and Vogel, E. F., Routledge and Kegan Paul, London.
6. Zijderveld, A. C. (1974), *The Abstract Society*, Pelican, London.
7. Jones, E. (1953), *Sigmund Freud*, Hogarth, London, vol. i, p. 269.
8. Holloway, F. (1979), *Freud, Biologist of the Mind*, Burnett Books, London.
9. Searles, H. (1979), 'The Patient as Therapist to his Analyst', in *Countertransference and Related Subjects*, International Universities Press, New York.
10. Winnicott, D. W. (1958), *Collected Papers*, Tavistock, London.
11. Milner, M. (1969), *The Hands of the Living God*, Hogarth, London.

9. The Teaching of Psychotherapy

When goodness is lost,
 there is kindness,
When kindness is lost,
 there is justice,
When justice is lost,
 there is ritual. – Lao-Tzu

Earlier in this book (Chapter 1) I suggested certain qualities which would seem to be important for anyone wishing to practise psychotherapy. The problem facing the teacher of psychotherapy is that he is required to recognize these qualities in a prospective pupil and to be able to foster them. This is a daunting feat. The relevant qualities – good judgement, patience, stamina, etc. – are not easily identifiable without considerable knowledge of the candidate. And it is even more difficult to know how to facilitate their growth. How, for instance, does one teach a person to be a good listener? Although we can never hope to find an omniscient committee capable of making the necessary assessments with much accuracy – let alone teaching wisdom – we would surely be wrong to throw up our hands in despair and abandon the whole idea of training psychotherapists. We do, however, need to recognize how extraordinarily difficult is the task and to have no illusions about the degree to which we fall short at present in its accomplishment.

One of the limitations of the present approach is the fact that current ideology leads us to seek the respectability of 'academic rigour'. We believe that our prospective students should be intellectuals, capable of mastering psychological theory, able to put down their experiences on paper and report them to their mentors in the framework of thought acceptable to them. We make their path easier – much easier – if they are doctors or psychiatrists. In so doing we exclude (at least from the higher ranks of the profession) all those who, however mature, gifted, and intuitive, lack, either by means of education or inclination, the opportunity to pass through the straight and narrow gate.

There are several reasons for the continued domination of psychotherapy by medicine. Although the contemporary physician relies much more on technology than in the past he is often still cast in the role of the wise man by his patients. They turn to him in their distress as if he were a psychotherapist, and it is difficult for both the medical profession and the public to abandon this image and to recognize psychotherapy as an autonomous discipline. Moreover, the widespread belief that psychological problems are organic in origin dies hard. In addition to these factors (although not entirely separate from them) there is, to be considered once again, the preoccupation of our society with certainty. We need to diagnose – to find a name for what is wrong with a 'sick' person. Since the time of Kraepelin psychiatrists have spent a great deal of time in research into an ever-increasing refinement of their system of labelling disease. This frantic pursuit could only be justified in the unlikely case of their being a multiplicity of 'mental illnesses' for which one could hope to find specific cures. One suspects, however, that the search derives in no small part from a wish for a comforting formula to explain disturbing phenomena – whether or not the formula brings us experientially closer to them.

One reason that is frequently put forward to justify the opinion that psychotherapists should be medically trained is the danger that a 'lay' therapist may fail to diagnose a physical illness which is causing his patient's distress. That such a danger exists is not in doubt; but it does not approach the degree estimated by the profession and certainly does not merit the decade of training required to make a physician. The non-medical therapist need only ensure that a patient has a consultation with a doctor before making the assumption that he requires no medical attention. In my own experience as a therapist I have found my medical knowledge to be only marginally useful. Ideally we should be competent in many fields which have a bearing on our work – but we have only one life. The emphasis on the primacy of medicine is seen in its full irony when we consider the fact that the organically orientated doctor makes frequent and sometimes appalling errors of treatment because of his failure to appreciate the psychogenic factors in illness, yet would ridicule the idea that a student be required to have six to ten years teaching in psychotherapy before being considered fit to train in medicine.

In one respect a training in psychiatry is clearly useful. The student will find himself in contact with very disturbed people for whose welfare he is responsible and he will inevitably gain some understanding of how such people think and behave. The same is, of course, true of the psychiatric nurse and social worker. It is, however, not all gain, for to set against it the conditions (as, for instance, a hospital ward where physical forms of treatment prevail) in which psychiatric patients can be observed may distort rather than facilitate the understanding of confusion and despair.

Even if it were accepted that psychotherapy should not be part of a medical empire there is no guarantee that its identity would be preserved for there are other disciplines – notably that of experimental psychology – to which the professional, in his search for intellectual security, may turn. He may thereby go out of the frying-pan into the fire. The only rational answer to this dilemma is the recognition that psychotherapy is a discipline in its own right and does not need to pay lip service to more established and respectable professions.

At the present time the teaching of psychotherapy is undertaken in organizations which promote theories and techniques markedly at variance with each other. It is, of course, not unusual for a discipline to be taught in different institutions, many or all of which have their own particular orientation. This is the case, for instance, with philosophy and history. Although some of these schools of thought will inevitably present a more realistic view of life than others, we usually find it acceptable that a graduate of one of them is justified in claiming the status of a master in the field of study. When it comes to psychotherapy, however, the matter is somewhat different. The graduate of a Freudian or Jungian institute does not call himself a psychotherapist (albeit with a special orientation) but a psychoanalyst (in the former case) and an analytical psychologist (in the latter case). This nomenclature betrays, I think, the fact that there is as yet no generally accepted coherent framework of thinking about psychotherapy and underlines the muddle of our present training facilities. Let us now take a closer look at current methods of teaching.

In Britain the two most prestigious organizations are probably the Freudian and Jungian training schemes. The largest, and by far the most influential, is the former. Other schemes have emerged which use the Freudian Institute as their model and offer a much more limited training, informed by Freudian theory, designed for those who do not aim at the heights of the profession.

In Freudian Institutes, in Britain, America, and elsewhere, the student (who is required to have a degree in medicine, psychology, or related subject) undertakes three main projects. Firstly, a personal analysis of a certain frequency and duration (usually five times weekly for a minimum of four years). Secondly, the psychotherapy of (usually) two patients under supervision. Thirdly, attendance at lectures and seminars over a period of four years or so. He may or may not be required to present a paper.

Leaving aside the criticisms I have already made about this kind of training (that the emphasis is on technique rather than relationship, that the focus is on the work of one thinker, and that the expense is crippling to all but the rich), what is to be said for and against such a regime?

Supervision of one's early work and discussion, in groups, with an experienced therapist are surely of value. Even more is to be said of personal therapy. Indeed, I would likely have the backing of most of my colleagues in suggesting that placing oneself in the hands of a therapist is by far the most important move a student can take if he wishes to understand the nature of the work and his own particular weaknesses and strengths in its performance.

So far so good. But when we come to consider the conditions under which the therapy (or, as it is usually called, the analysis) is undertaken there are three questions that we need to ask.

Firstly, should we *require* a student to subject himself to therapy? Before answering in the affirmative we do well to remember that most therapists feel much more optimistic about a patient who comes out of an inner desire to change rather than from a recommendation by others that he undertake the therapy.

Secondly, should we prescribe the frequency and duration of the student's therapy, in view of the fact that such decisions can only be realistically made by the two people concerned and will vary enormously from case to case?

Thirdly, does not the routine reporting of the student's 'progress' to the training committee destroy the (immeasurably valuable) confidentiality of the therapeutic relationship?

To continue our investigation of current training programmes we must now turn to the manner and style of the teaching. What happens in the therapy will depend (except in so far as the above considerations impinge upon it) on the personality and methods of the particular therapist. But what of the nature of the regime as a whole?

Methods of education, at all levels and for all ages, have been the subject of much controversy in recent decades, and the matter is by no means settled. It would seem, however, that those of us who see psychotherapy as a means of promoting the growth of autonomy and creative individuality must take the ideas of Rousseau, Pestalozzi, Froebel, and Dewey very seriously. Moreover, since students of psychotherapy are – if suitably selected – capable of taking a great deal of responsibility for themselves, we should provide them with a training which gives maximum attention to their self-determination. Consequently, we should question the value of teaching organizations which set out to instruct students of psychotherapy in a body of received knowledge, which lay down rigid requirements on courses of study, and which have the conventional structure of traditional hierarchical institutions (with their accompanying inflexibility). Yet these schemes remain in the ascendant – and I believe they do so because of the excessive concern with control and security which (as I have stressed throughout this book) is a mark of our present culture.

When in trouble we seek someone to trust. He may be known to us personally, he may be recommended by a friend, or he may be a person of status – approved by a respected organization. We fear the charlatan: the man who publicly claims a competence he does not possess, who may deceive people into a trust that is without any justification. That society should attempt to protect us from the charlatan is surely right and proper. But, in relation to psychotherapy, there are certain problems about the protective measures taken.

Those psychotherapists who consider their profession to be a science are in a much more vulnerable academic position than, say, surgeons or physicists. It is difficult for them to demonstrate the validity of their results or to counteract the charge that their work and training lacks rigour. In the attempt to overcome an embarrassing sense of inferiority, psychotherapeutic training schemes prescribe ever-increasing demands that their students show that they have applied themselves to a rigorous discipline of some kind. The advantage of these measures is that they deter those who seek a soft option. The disadvantage is that students may be subjected to inappropriate and confusing tasks in order to present a respectable face to the public and to fellow-professionals.

The current moves, in Britain, towards a Register of Psychotherapists adds urgency to these questions. To my mind, such a register would probably do more harm than good. If it does come about it would be wise to ensure that its power is limited to excluding those professionals whose moral behaviour falls short of that which the public has a right to enjoy and to make the requirement that a practitioner, if asked by a prospective client, give an honest answer about his training and experience. It would, in this event, still remain open to certain training organizations, or other independent bodies, to make available a list of those practitioners in whom they place confidence.

One of the reasons for the present muddle in attempts to discover a place in society for the psychotherapist is, I think, the fact that it is so difficult to find realistic criteria for the measurement of psycho-therapeutic ability. A comparison with art may help in understand-ing the problem.

Let us imagine a child who shows an aptitude for and interest in art and subsequently studies at a college of art where he learns a great deal, passes an examination, and is awarded a degree. If he were now to seek a place in education or commerce his degree would be an important passport. But if his ambition is to make and sell objects of beauty, then (leaving aside the vicissitudes of fashion and his ability to advertise) he will be judged on the artistic merits of his products. People will buy what he makes if they like it irrespec-tive of any certificate of competence he may or may not possess.

The psychotherapist's work is, to my mind, more like that of the artist or craftsman than the scientist. He is engaged with divergent rather than convergent problems: his product is unique. But there are two differences when the question of assessment arises. Firstly, his product is more elusive than that of the artist. It is not there, to behold, in the public eye. Secondly, because his efforts are directed towards people's health rather than their aesthetic sensibilities, he is – at least in our society as opposed to, say, Eastern Europe – considered more dangerous than the artist: bad art may be deplored but the 'quack' is feared as a menace. As a consequence of these differences society seeks to control the psychotherapist by requiring of him a certificate of competence whereas (in this country and provided it is not deemed obscene) the artist may create what he chooses, and the public may themselves choose his products on the basis of their own perception and judgement. Psychotherapy falls between two stools: a certificate is of very uncertain value yet the public have no ready means of estimating the worth of a prac-titioner.

Our hope must lie in a radical change in the conception of psychotherapy, and this change has much in common with that required in our thinking about the training, practice, and organization of other professions (e.g. education) which depend for their vitality on the quality of the personal relationships between those who seek help and those who seek to provide. I believe that there is still sufficient dissatisfaction in our present society, among both professionals and public, to give hope of a major change in our attitude to healing, despite the fact that so many radical ventures of recent years have either petered out because of opposition or attracted too many of those whose interest is merely in the novel and fashionable.

To set against the increasing impersonal specialization of our times there is a powerful current of opinion, with a respectable pedigree in European thought dating back to the Greeks, through which is expressed the recognition of the crippling grip of bureaucratic and compartmentalized living. Those who belong to this movement find themselves, *faute de mieux*, using words like 'whole', 'real', 'personal', 'human', 'spiritual', etc., in an attempt to delineate their protest – words which, because they so easily lend themselves to facile, sentimental, and woolly modes of thought, draw derision from opponents to this view. And action based on these beliefs is similarly vulnerable to confusion and misunderstanding.

The traditional, hierarchical organizations that I have discussed above are, of course, not the only contenders in the field. In the past two decades an increasing number of counter-movements, most of which originated in the United States, have emerged. I refer to 'alternative therapies': Gestalt, Bio-energetics, Clinical Theology, Primal Scream, T-groups, etc. A detailed critique of these methods lies outside the scope of this book for they are focused on group rather than individual therapy. However, despite the valuable insights gained in this work and the merit that it can bring psychotherapeutic help to those who need it and cannot find it, these movements have serious disadvantages. Firstly, the emphasis on technique remains; secondly, there appears to be little recognition of the fact that, in the matter of psychological healing, the success of short-cut methods is often more apparent than real and dramatization all too easy; and thirdly, in place of true equality, there tends to be an idealization of charismatic figures. (There may be certain differences in English and American vulnerabilities here. Whereas the Americans are more able to undermine the inhibitions of formality and protocol they seem less able to spot the false note in much of the current psychological writings on precipitate intimacy.)

Although, for the reasons given, I cannot entirely share the philosophy of the Encounter Movement, it is clear that the kind of training which follows logically from the views put forward in this book has much in common with all those thinkers – within or outside the psychotherapeutic field – who seek an alternative structure to the dominant pattern of professional teaching and practice. A rather more extreme line than my own is taken by the Dutch psychoanalyst Bondewijn Chabot, who, in a paper entitled 'The Right to Care for Each Other', argues powerfully for the *abolition* of the psychotherapeutic profession. Chabot believes that:

. . . an unobserved and very subtle process of erosion is taking place in regard to 'the care for each other'. In this process at least one necessary condition for this kind of care is being undermined: the confidence that through one's life experiences, one can develop a specific, natural gift and inclination to a degree of high competence. From the (hesitant beginnings of) environmental legislation we know that interference with a condition that is essential to a certain desirable development can have juridical consequences. Though (lack of) care for our natural environment is currently receiving some juridical attention, an analogous approach to our social environment is still lacking. The reason for this may lie, I hope, in the fact that the erosion of the conditions for real care in the context of personal relationships is not progressing at as fast a rate as I now think.[1]

In spite of recognizing Chabot as someone whose thought is close to my own, I think he underestimates the value of the professional stance. In turning to the professional we have the assurance that he is a dedicated worker who has given much time and effort to learning a technique which at least he believes is relevant to our predicament, and who, because he has not been excommunicated by his fellows, is presumably someone with a sense of responsibility. Even if his training has been inappropriate he has spent time with troubled people and is likely to have learnt something of their ways. And the status which society gives him enables him to organize situations in which people can come together in the presence of a person whose authority and tact make possible a fruitful outcome. He can pour oil on troubled waters. Earlier (Chapter 3) I indicated some of the advantages which the professional psychotherapeutic situation has over that which exists with a sympathetic and wise friend.

In recent years, in an attempt to confront this dilemma, I have worked with a group of people who – partly out of their philosophy of living and partly out of practical need – sought to turn themselves into counsellors or psychotherapists by means of the 'de-schooling' model.

Until moving, in the last couple of years, to the city where I now work, I lived and practised in a country town where psychotherapists were thin on the ground and the London training centres a two-hour journey away. In this area a number of us joined together to create a training set-up using the available local (non-institutional) sources. We met weekly. I was the only experienced psychotherapist in the group, but arrangements were made for therapists to come from London and give seminars. Formality of any kind was minimal; there was no curriculum; each topic was approached from the point of naïve and personal experience; everything was questioned; emphasis was placed on practical experience, personal therapy, mutual supervision, and flexibility of thought.

On one occasion the group combined in the treatment of a 'schizophrenic' patient who had refused to go to hospital and had no money (one member taking on the task of individual therapy), with a result that was as rewarding as anything I have witnessed in my career.

It would, I think, be out of place to present a detailed account here of the problems which the group faced and their attempts to solve them. The two most obvious ones were: firstly, the undue weight likely to be given (however much we strove to avoid this) to the only experienced psychotherapist available for regular discussion; and secondly, the fact that members had to relinquish the recognition that is usually given to a 'graduate' of a comparable group organized on conventional lines. What I wish to suggest is that such a group can be a viable alternative to the normal career structure in spite of enormous practical difficulties, can do so without relinquishing rigour, will promote autonomy and creative thinking more readily than conventional training schemes; and to record that the cohesiveness of this particular group appeared to depend more upon a shared philosophy of living than on any other factor. From my experience with this and other (very different) groups and my work as a psychotherapist, I would like to make certain comments about a desirable training.

While the practice of psychotherapy requires dedication, effort, and teaching, yet the qualities which are of most significance in one's capacity to do the work cannot be learned from books or a course of training in the way one could, for instance, learn clinical pathology. It has not the specificity of knowledge and skill that is usually attributed to it and in judging the competence of a therapist we should therefore not depart radically from the way in which we judge anybody's capacity to help. More important than his specialized knowledge is the therapist's presentation of himself in the therapeutic setting. Therefore a training should start from the recognition that a learned technique not only cannot substitute for a more elemental capacity to heal but may actually inhibit this capacity: that it should be less a course of instruction than an attempt to increase an individual's unique capacity to help.

The form a training in psychotherapy may take should not, I believe, be precisely laid down before the event. It will depend on the people involved and the circumstances; and it should be allowed to grow. The following suggestions and comments are therefore of a provisional nature, and refer to a possible teaching set-up I would regard as appropriate to the kind of work I describe in this book.

1. It would be initiated by a group of people whose basic orientation to living, learning, and healing was similar. Some of these people would be teachers, some students.

2. The structure of the group would not be hierarchical in the traditional manner.*

3. The main aim of the group would be the enquiry into and teaching of ways in which disturbed people can be helped in various situations. Although the kind of group I myself have in mind would focus on 'individual psychotherapy', other groups may focus on different situations or even on the study of the elements common to all helping endeavours.

4. What is taught is a function of the way it is taught: personal psychotherapy cannot be adequately taught in a setting that departs radically from the philosophical beliefs that inform our work. If we believe that individual psychotherapy is a process by means of

* For a discussion of the illogicality of hierarchical systems see (among the many writings on the subject) *Education for Power* by Andrew Czartoryski, Davis-Poynter, London, 1975.

which two people, of equal worth, struggle together on a path with no signpost, relying for the most part on their ordinary human virtues and capacities, the difference being that one of them has acted before as guide and assistant to other people on other paths, then one must teach psychotherapy in the same way.

5. It is to be expected that students will vary considerably in ability, dedication, and opportunity to pursue studies, and therefore there would be no 'course' in the sense of a procedure lasting a certain length of time. Consequently no *uniform* qualification, certificate of competence, or record of attendance would be appropriate. However, in an honest atmosphere students whose work appeared to be futile would be discouraged by the group from practising and those who eventually leave the group may apply to it for references in the same way that an ex-employee of a business firm would do.

6. If I were a teacher in a group which focused on individual therapy I would make clear my belief that the two most important factors in any training are firstly, personal therapy; secondly, being with disturbed people; and thirdly, personal supervision of early work. And I would regard it as essential that no report is required by anybody from the student's therapist.

7. Finally, a word about the selection of students. Selection of candidates is not always left to a training institute, for some select themselves: those who have such a determination to do the work and are so able at it that they will become psychotherapists provided no law is passed which prohibits them. A teacher is fortunate when such a person asks for his help. But most of those who wish to practise therapy need the support, encouragement, and legitimization of a psychotherapeutic training scheme, and in these cases a judgement has to be made. The selectors must do their best to recognize wisdom. One dilemma is the fact that, although to practise psychotherapy with reasonable competence a person should not be too 'sick', nevertheless the experience of psychological disturbance is of enormous help in understanding those in anguish. When I consider those colleagues whose work I greatly value, I find that most of them turned to psychotherapy in the first place out of their own personal need. And when we look at the great figures of the past we find the same: the 'creative illness' through which both Freud and Jung passed have been described by Ellenberger[2] and others. At best selection is a hazardous

procedure. Due respect should be given to both the wishes of the group as a whole and the weight carried by the judgement of experienced practitioners.

In order for the kind of scheme I have indicated to emerge, a number of psychotherapists would need to come together and lend their experience in such a way that someone could use it to enhance his own unique capacity to help others; and a sufficient number of students be found with the kind of perspective that would enable them to benefit from such a regime. A balance would have to be struck between these ideals and the need to take account of the fact that students will be required to justify their training to a society that, for the most part, idealizes formal, oversimplified, and quantified evidence of training. I am not suggesting that such a compromise would be easy but that we should attempt to find one which involves less of a capitulation to the impersonal, centralized ideology of our time than those training schemes which currently command respect.

With increasing availability of psychotherapeutic help in the community – from the ordinary citizen to practitioners of experience – the focus on 'crisis intervention' rather than 'hospitalization' would be greater, and expense saved on inefficient treatment and the overprescribing of drugs could be put to psychotherapeutic use. Moreover, the acceptance of the fact that psychotherapy is not as far removed from other pursuits as is commonly supposed could lessen the gap between it and those disciplines (such as education) with comparable aims, and increase the contribution it can make to the critique of the dominant contemporary picture of ourselves and the world we live in. It can do this by bringing to the debate what can be understood when two people meet in favourable conditions with a sense of equality and an absence of drama, and both explore the possibilities of mutual trust – free, for a while, from some of the limitations which our culture imposes on those who want to come close to each other. I do not refer to a reorganization of the social services in order to bring help to those who need it – although there is room for improvement in this sphere – but a basic change in our conception of the nature of healing.

The attitude of those of us who think in this way is a matter of temperament and strategy. We may work quietly – individually or in groups – in the hope that some of our beliefs may spread to others. Or, fearing danger to our aims by the increasing tendency of society towards excessive impersonality, we may, as I have done in this book, and as others will do in their various ways, speak out in an attempt to stem the tide and put the case for the personal.

References

1. Chabot, B. (1979), 'The Right to Care for Each Other and its Silent Erosion', published in Dutch, *Tijdschrift Voor Psychotherapie*, 5. 199.
2. Ellenberger, H. F. (1970), *The Discovery of the Unconscious*, Allen Lane, London.

10. Postscript

Hope is forever stealing the little time life allotts us, and
our last dawn overtakes us with so many dreams unfulfilled.
– Julius Polyaenus of Sardinia (trans. I. F. Stone)

Enthusiasts – among whom I count myself – speak readily of
the satisfactions of their pursuits, and minimize the frustrations,
failures, disappointments, and heartache. In this book I have been
in danger not only of smoothing over the raggedness and useless-
ness of some of my work but, because of my particular theoretical
orientation, of giving the impression that psychotherapy is easy.
Such an impression would be very wrong. Rather I believe it to be a
path which is hard and stony along which each of us will travel
according to his talent, dedication, stamina, and luck.

The reader will, no doubt, have made his own judgement of my
work from the style as well as the content of the presentation and
will perhaps have gained some idea what it is like to be with me in
the consulting room. But I have made no deliberate attempt to
convey what the work means to me, why I do it, and the price I pay
for doing it. This sort of thing cannot, of course, be measured
quantitatively. Life is not easy for most of us either because of harsh
circumstances or inner conflicts, and work, in our driven, competitive, and lonely society, is often stressful. The hazards of
psychotherapy are in many ways similar to those of comparable
occupations: we are, at least in this country, not obviously more or
less privileged or at risk than those in other professions.

I have little to tell my colleagues about the pain of psychotherapy
for we are all in the same boat – although I sometimes feel we could
share our feelings more unreservedly than we usually do. This
chapter is therefore avowedly a postscript, to be read separately
from the rest of the book, and is addressed to those who have not
themselves experienced the sadness intrinsic to the practice of
psychotherapy. But the discontinuity with what has gone before is
not absolute for much that I have criticized in psychoanalytical
theory derives, I believe, from attempts to escape from pain and to
divert our attention from the fact of sadness to its explanation.

Unwelcome emotions are bound to arise during any long-term
relationship. It is discomforting to face continued exposure to the
hate, confusion, misery, rigidity, or dependence of those whom one

must try to tolerate and even attempt to heal. Ultimate failure is particularly hard to bear. Even after taking into consideration the neurotic guilt and the hurt pride of performance which few psychotherapists can avoid, there remains an elemental grief in watching someone with whom one has become intimate destroy his life in one way or another. At times my contact with patients has shaken me to the depths of my being, provoked me to act towards them in destructive and shameful ways and has, I suspect, made me physically ill; and, in my earlier years of practice, before I became able to defend myself better, has drained me of some of my energy and patience which I now feel were due to my family and friends. Indeed, I have even had the thought – although I do not believe it to be justified – that it is asking too much of one person to be both a therapist and a parent. Of the pressures which bear upon the therapist, the most fearsome, I believe, is that of dependence. I used to think that a tendency to overconscientiousness on my part accounted for the weight of it but, having heard colleagues speak of this pressure, and remembering, with some remorse, the burden I must unthinkingly have placed on my own therapist, I regard it as, to some extent, an occupational hazard. I am supported in this thought by the fact that a certain number of people in the caring professions in therapy with me who have wished to become thera-pists have decided against it after realizing the emotional impact of a *long-term* commitment. I can sympathize with them. Sometimes when a patient is referred to me I experience a sinking feeling as I intuit-ively recognize the extent of the caring being asked for. The thera-pist has, of course, a legitimate means of protecting himself from the emotions provoked in him by the patient. He can recognize that they are often stimulated more by the patient's fantasy or reality-testing rather than actual need – and the art of therapy is, in part, to accept the distortions without cynicism. But this is easier said than done. Feelings of anguish do not necessarily subside on receipt of insight. Moreover, how experienced and wise does one have to be to make certain judgements as to the degree to which it is neces-sary to accede to the patient's apparent needs? I know of a psychoanalyst who telephoned one of his patients every night for a year or more in the belief that this symbolic equivalent of being tucked into bed by a parent was vital to her recovery. Was he right? And, if so, how many of us would be as confident and willing to go to such lengths? Unless one is gifted beyond the normal I believe the making of such judgements is severely taxing. Some of the most painful experiences I have suffered are occasions when I have given my heart to a patient only to find that the sincerity of my behaviour had been understood by him as a triumph of his manipulative power.

There is, to my mind, no doubt of the fact that many, and probably most, psychotherapists are drawn to their work because they themselves grew up in unhappy families and early conceived a desire to repair the hurt in others. This is no cause for alarm unless the urge to heal is carried to a compulsive degree – unless the therapist cannot tolerate failure, is consumed by guilt towards his patients, overprotects them as a consequence, and is unduly sensitive to the charge of failing to make them happy. This is certainly a hazard in my own case. Although I do not take the cynical view that a sensitivity to the needs of others is necessarily derived from an inauthentic desire to be a saint, the dangers to the therapist of narcissistic indulgence in his position are clearly great. Firstly, he has to remain unaffected by the idealization which patients, in their need, bestow upon him. Secondly, he knows that in a real way he is a crucially important person to many people. And thirdly, the pain of failure, when it occurs, is so devastating that he is tempted to buttress himself against it by denying the limitations of his competence.

The distinction between a sensitivity which permits the therapist to tune in to others and the sensitivity (usually referred to as *over*-sensitivity) which has its basis in an undue preoccupation with one's self-image is a narrow but crucial one. I sometimes feel that not only is the main aim of therapy to reduce the patient's narcissism but that one's career as a therapist is one long struggle against the same afflictions. To the extent that I have succeeded in my own struggle I have become more able to help people. And it is likely that the writing of this book – which can be thought of as a plea for humility in both theory and practice – has been, in part, engendered by this fight. But, let me hasten to add, I do not write from the comfortable position of the one who believes he has won a notable victory. Although I am now more successful in my work than earlier I can still fail through lack of humility. Narcissism may reveal itself in a controlled attitude of paternalism and a complacent assumption that the 'rules' of therapy are above reproach or in a disproportionate reaction to criticism. I will give an example of the latter.

Some years ago a middle-aged man came to see me who was

married and successful in his work but deeply anxious and unhappy. He had been to several psychotherapists previously but had apparently gained no help. It is not, I think, important in this context to relate the details of his life story. What is relevant is the way he behaved to me. I found him quite an engaging person to talk to but as time went on he became more and more reproachful about what he referred to as my 'coldness'. Such an accusation, whether justified or not, is of course familiar to all therapists, but in this case there was an unhappy combination of affairs. Because I was moved by his real anguish I could not remain indifferent; his persuasive catalogue of my failings carried a conviction greater than I usually encounter; and, finally, I am more vulnerable than many to a persistent and powerful condemnation for being 'cold' because I have earlier been subjected to this criticism by my mother (for reasons which I now can understand as part of a family pattern). In time his attitude got under my skin and I was provoked to shouting at him in my fury. He took this as a final rejection and refused to see me again, writing me a letter of extreme bitterness. I think, on reflection, that it would have been better to accept my limitations and terminate the therapy much sooner.

I suggested earlier that, because of both the nature of the task and the type of neurotic urges which frequently have a bearing on the choice of professions, the dependence of patients is often the most hazardous ordeal which a psychotherapist has to face. But it is not without its rewards. Let me end with an account of an interchange with a patient whose dependence I have at times found difficult to accept.

Sonia is a woman of my own age, whom I have been seeing for about fifteen years. She lives in a country on the other side of Europe, and, because her opinion of psychiatric practice there is low, she travels to England every year or so to have a few weeks of daily sessions with me. During her stay she regresses to a state of dependence and engages in a period of intense effort. How she manages to pull herself together and return each time to her very demanding work is a wonder to me. I shall not describe her history except to say that her brother died when she was two months old, her mother fell into a state of profound grief, and Sonia seemed to have had a childhood of hopeless misery. On the second night of her recent therapy she had the following dream: 'An old woman was emptying a bag of clothes, distributing them at random.'

We had already noted her present state of disorganization in England following a long period of hard work at home and we felt that the dream was a representation of this state. In referring to the dream again Sonia use the word 'rags' instead of clothes and continued: 'I am empty and worthless inside'. My response was to say that ragged clothes can be colourful, and to comment that the term 'ragamuffin' conjured up for me an exciting, wild, free person.

'No,' she said, sadly; 'These were grey rags.'

Although I could argue in defence of my optimistic comment about the dream, it would seem that I was trying to avoid the impact of her misery.

That night I slept badly and started the day feeling rather anxious without obvious reason. Sonia was my second patient. She came looking very depressed and withdrawn. I now remembered the impact she had sometimes had on me in previous years.

'I am so very tired,' she said, in a low voice. I myself soon began to feel depressed and inadequate, and Sonia noticed.

'Why do you hide from me?' she asked. 'Why are you so far away? Are you depressed? I feel so withdrawn myself – I suppose I make you withdrawn.' This was spoken in a despairing rather than angry voice.

I told her that I was tired, that I had been very busy the previous day. I did not tell her (rightly or wrongly) that I was now beginning to wonder whether my disturbed night was in anticipation of her depression. I was confused, evasive, and felt like someone trying to keep afloat.

Sonia continued, 'You *must* be withdrawn for me. I make you so. Perhaps so that I can again experience my mother's withdrawal. I turned my body to her and she gave me nothing . . . can you stand it? Do you hate me? Do you despise me?'

'No.'

'I take everything, I must drain you. How do you manage to survive patients like me? Doesn't it exhaust you?'

'Yes, I sometimes feel that people ask more than I can give but I wouldn't do another job for the world.'*

'Say that again . . . please.'

I repeated my statement.

Sonia looked relieved. 'Thank you for saying that.'

---

* Although this is near the truth I believe I overstated the case in order to reassure Sonia.

At the end of the session she said, 'Thank you for not avoiding the difficulties.'

The next day Sonia told me that after our meeting she had thought: 'If someone from my country wanted to see an analyst in England would I suggest Peter Lomas? No. There would be no point. I shall have eaten him all up.'

The subsequent events of Sonia's visit give an indication of one of the hazards – of quite a different nature – which also besets the psychotherapist.

Although there was no repetition of the crisis that I felt within myself, Sonia continued to be depressed. One day when she was silent and aware only of loneliness and emptiness I could find no sensible thing to say. I told her so and said that the only thing which came to mind was the wish that she meet my wife and daughter.

Sonia, knowing that my daughter is artistic, has said that she would be welcome to stay with her and look at the art of her own country. I had mentioned this invitation to my daughter a few days previously and she had been delighted with the idea, although in practice it would be difficult for her to make the journey. My wife, who was in the room at the time, said, 'Does the invitation include me?'

I repeated this conversation to Sonia, adding that I felt that the three of them had a similar outlook on life and would understand each other.

Sonia was moved by this. 'That makes you feel real.' Her depression lifted and we talked at length about the meaning of it all: of the child who needs a mother who is also a friend, of the possibility of my joining the party visiting her home, of the risks and vulnerabilities on both sides if we were to do this. It was a new thought to her that the risks on my side would be comparable to her own. The conversation was a relief to us and we laughed at ourselves.

I do not know at this point whether the visit will take place. I am aware of, yet afraid of, a potential friendship. There are not many people whose continued warmth and respect I would value as much as Sonia's.

When things go well between a therapist and a patient it is likely that they will grow to enjoy each other's company. If this occurs they may have to accept limitations imposed by the conditions of therapy on a potential rich friendship. In many situations of life there are temptations to cross barriers which, if one succumbed to them, would prove destructive; but the intensity of the therapeutic encounter ensures that these temptations are strong.

The ending of therapy may be painful not only for the patient but for the therapist. The question arises: should they part and not see each other again? If they decide to continue meeting, what are the hazards? When two people have gained something from each other in a special and unusual setting there is no guarantee that the mutuality would be possible in other circumstances, and they have to gauge whether the risk is worth taking. Therapy is, in this respect as in so many others, not dissimilar to parenthood. There is a time when it is better for a child to leave home and perhaps there is a time when it is better for a patient to leave the person who has cared for him – however much they may have grown to enjoy each other. And the acceptance of this can be painful. Many of the people whom I have come most to admire and like in my life have been patients, yet, in those cases where we have changed the relationship into a simple friendship, the process has often been fraught with problems, not only because the patient has found it difficult to abandon his dependent feelings, but because it is frustrating for both people to lose the degree of intimacy to which they have become accustomed.

How can one find a way among these hazards? Once again I recommend that we turn to daily living for our understanding. There is a limit to the degree of emotional commitment of which we are capable. Like the porcupines that seek closeness for warmth yet must not get too near to the prickles of their fellows, we, in so far as we are healthy, discover the optimum distance – which varies from time to time and person to person – from our relatives and friends. And so it must be in therapy if the practitioner is to survive.

Index